The Social Construction of Community Nursing

Anne Kelly and Anthea Symonds

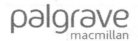
palgrave
macmillan

First published 2003 by
PALGRAVE MACMILLAN
Houndmills, Basingstoke, Hampshire RG21 6XS and
175 Fifth Avenue, New York, N.Y. 10010
Companies and representatives throughout the world

PALGRAVE MACMILLAN is the global academic imprint of the Palgrave Macmillan division of St. Martin's Press, LLC and of Palgrave Macmillan Ltd. Macmillan® is a registered trademark in the United States, United Kingdom and other countries. Palgrave is a registered trademark in the European Union and other countries.

ISBN 0–333–75006–3 paperback

This book is printed on paper suitable for recycling and made from fully managed and sustained forest sources.

A catalogue record for this book is available from the British Library.

10 9 8 7 6 5 4 3 2 1
12 11 10 09 08 07 06 05 04 03

Printed and bound in Great Britain by
Creative Print & Design (Wales), Ebbw Vale

To all community nurses,
past, present and future

Contents

List of Figures and Tables

Figures

Tables

Foreword

Health care systems across the world are confronted by the problem of ever-increasing demands for services against a background of constraints on the resources available to provide them. The problem represents a major headache for those at all levels of policy-making, decision-making and commissioning services and for those at the forefront of service provision and delivery. The need to ensure that limited resources are channelled into effective interventions has provided additional impetus to the drive towards evidence-based practice, while at the same time endeavouring to reduce levels of inequalities which exist in terms of provision and health status. The notion of evidence-based practice, with its emphasis not only on how health professionals practise, but also on what they practise, has been one of the factors which have resulted in the appraisal of the roles and responsibilities of health care professionals. In addition, the social status of health care professionals in society has shifted following high profile media cases, which have seriously undermined public confidence in the health care professions.

At the same time it is becoming increasingly apparent that health professionals must learn to increasingly work in partnership relationships with other agencies and members of local communities to promote health effectively. Community involvement in health through such partnerships has been widely advocated, but translating intention into practice is complex and represents a challenge for all the stakeholders involved in the change process. Such partnership arrangements require a transformation of the professional role from protagonist to partner, and the patient–client role from passive recipient to partner. These partnership approaches have considerable merit in health care systems that emphasise active involvement and self-care actions of individuals and families to maintain health and prevent disease, and the role of community nurses within such situations has particular significance. Partnership approaches and the role of community nurses are also important in situations involving underserved, vulnerable, ethnic minority and other socially excluded groups in society. For too long, professionals and policy-makers have relegated these groups to passive roles in health decision-making and action, with health inequalities providing vivid testimony of such neglect.

Furthermore, it is generally accepted that the relationship between expenditure on health care services and the health status of a population is not directly proportional. It is far too simplistic to argue that in order to improve the health of the nation and reduce inequalities, additional resources need to be channelled into health care services. After all, the USA is one of the least healthy of the wealthy nations of the world, despite spending some 14 per cent of its GDP on health care while Japan, which spends about 7 per cent of its GDP on health care, is one of the healthiest. Understanding the state of health within a community and differences between communities requires thinking about the wider determinants of health, which again highlights the pivotal role of community nurses in facilitating improvements in the health of such communities and the wider aspects of social welfare.

This book charts the historical developments that have occurred in the roles of community nurses, and argues strongly that the profession needs to embrace traditional and contemporary models of nursing and social care if it is to continue to make a significant contribution to the health and wellbeing of society, in the light of current health and social policy developments.

Dr Ceri Phillips
Reader

Acknowledgements

The authors would like to thank the following people whose work has contributed to the content of this book; Angela Jones, Stephanie Jones, Janice Lewis, Gail Mooney and Greg and Sue Summer.

Their hard work has provided information about current situations in community nursing. Also we would like to acknowledge the administrative support of Joyce Owen, CHEPS, School of Health Science, The University of Wales Swansea, without whose help this book would not have materialised.

List of Acronyms

BMA	British Medical Association
BMJ	British Medical Journal
CETHV	Council for Education and Training of Health Visitors
COHSE	Confederation of Health Service Employees
CPHVA	Community Practitioners and Health Visitors Association
CPN	Community Psychiatric Nurse
DoH	Department of Health
DHSS	Department of Health and Social Security
GDP	Gross Domestic Product
GNC	General Nursing Council
GP	General Practitioner
HEA	Health Education Authority
HVA	Health Visitors Association
LCC	London County Council
NASW	National Association of Social Workers
NAYIC	National Association of Young People in Care
NHS	National Health Service
NHSME	National Health Service Management Executive
PHC	Primary Health Care
PHG	Primary Health Group
PSU	Pacifist Service Unit
RCN	Royal College of Nursing
SEU	Social Exclusion Unit
UKCC	United Kingdom Central Council for Nursing, Midwifery and Health Visiting
UN	United Nations
WHO	World Health Organisation

PART I

THE CONSTRUCTION OF COMMUNITY NURSING

Introduction

Part I of our book seeks to construct an understanding of the social meaning of community-based nursing. There are many questions regarding this particular branch of nursing: What do we mean by community nursing? Why did it emerge? Who were community nurses and who are they today? What was its original purpose and has that changed? What does it feel like to be a community nurse today? What makes community-based nursing so distinctive from hospital nursing?

The most obvious and fundamental difference is of course the *site* of practice. This is nursing practice removed from its institutional base – the hospital. It involves different social relationships not just between the nurse and the community but also within the hierarchical power structure of the health service. Community nursing can in many ways be seen as 'real' nursing in the real world. But the site and everyday practices of health visiting, district nursing, school nursing and mental nursing were founded upon contradictions and these still remain:

Contradictions of *site*:
- Public health/Private home
- Collective provision/Individual targeting

Community nurses operate within territory which is owned by the client. This in itself marks it out from hospital-based nursing and sets up problems for the negotiation of power relations. The collective element in much of public health, the universalism of health visiting, for example, contrasts with the targeting of *individuals and families* for attention.

The contradictions within *practice* can be defined as:
- Care/Education
- Support/Control

All community nursing contains within it the educative function. The delivery of care is connected to the delivery of knowledge which will enable the patient

1

or carer to manage their health or care in a more efficient way. Equally, support for individuals and families is connected to a degree of control over their lives wherein they enter into a 'settlement' with community nurses and in exchange for care delivery they themselves become the subject of surveillance. These contradictions of site and practice were inherent within the construction of all branches of community nursing. This section does not attempt to chronicle a history of community nursing but to place its construction against a background of the concerns, discourses and policies which created a specific role for each branch. The underlying contention is that nursing in the site of the community was constructed to fulfil a specific role which overtly was within health and social care delivery, but which also was in the vanguard of the everyday administration of social order.

Governmentality

In order to clarify this argument we must utilise the work of Foucault, and other writers who also have used his theories on power and administration, to illuminate the meaning of the power of medicine and allied discourses in the construction of health services of modern states.

The work of Foucault has been widely used within studies of medicine and nursing but Foucault did not directly apply his theories to the development of health policies. Nevertheless, it is possible to understand the increased role of state intervention in the implementation of public health policies, the development of medical power and of health education policies within his theoretical framework.

Firstly, Foucault saw power as existing within *relationships* and *sites* rather than as a macro structure based in all the institutions of a Capitalist society as Marxists had previously defined it. In his study of the emergence of psychiatric medicine and the institutionalisation and objectification of 'madness' (Foucault 1973), he saw power as 'embodied in the day to day practices of the medical profession' (Turner 1997). This view of power relations as existing in everyday practices between people and especially between health professionals and clients must be placed within his theory of the necessity for a system of social order.

Foucault saw social order as the principal problem faced by the emerging modern and industrialising states from the end of the eighteenth century. New government apparatuses of administration were needed to exercise a *discipline* over a newly mobile and potentially out-of-control population. Mechanisms for the control and administration of populations Foucault defined as 'governmentality' (Foucault 1991). One of the most important elements of this mechanism was the increasing control exercised over human bodies. This control was illustrated in the new sciences of criminology and psychiatry and manifested in the building of a new design of institutions including prisons, hospitals and schools. A clear illustration of this can be seen in the design of the Nightingale wards with the nurses' station placed so that all the beds can be observed from one single point. Schoolrooms were designed with an elevated stage at one end from which the one teacher could observe all the desks. Prisons were designed to enable the few to exercise surveillance over the many via the rounded panopticon which allowed for constant visibility. Another, more covert, illustration of this form of control and discipline over the body was, of course, exercised by the new knowledge and power of bio-medicine. Writers such as Armstrong (1983, 1995), have argued that this control exercised by 'surveillance medicine' was a feature of Britain and other European states from the nineteenth century onwards.

The legislation on public health in Britain during the nineteenth and early twentieth century is evidence that a new form of administration was being developed. The health of the population became an increasing object of concern to governments and through public health measures a degree of order and discipline was maintained. But this concern over the health of the population was only possible because of increasing knowledge of populations which was constructed via the collection of statistics on mortality, especially infant mortality, and changing theories on causation of disease.

The medical profession, which was legitimised by the state in the middle of the nineteenth century, played a leading role in the construction of the body as a site of discipline as disease was located within the individual anatomy. But this stage followed the acceptance by government that it was responsible for providing the conditions for good health and the cessation of epidemics in the legislation on sewage disposal, clean water, housing and pollution control. Armstrong (1993) has defined the stages of public health during the nineteenth century as developing from quarantine involving a separation of spaces and policed by state regulations to the separation of bodies and ideas of personal hygiene which were policed by health professionals. But the idea that individuals were in some way responsible for their own health could only be possible when the structural conditions were in place. As Osborne has noted about this development of concepts and definitions of health:

> One moves very quickly from the idea of health as being a right of citizenship to that of health being a duty of citizenship. (Osborne 1997:181)

When we look at the progression of health policies in Britain from the nineteenth to the end of the twentieth century, we can detect this change in the relationship between the government, the citizen and health.

But to return to the Foucauldian concept of the exercise of power as being embodied in everyday practice. The role of community nursing as a mechanism for order now becomes central to this idea of the 'governmentality' of society being carried out by everyday practices in health care. Nelson has applied this argument to the case of Ireland, and argued that nurses were 'in the front line in the techniques of pastoral government in the nineteenth century' (Nelson 1997:6). This view of nursing and especially community-based nursing as being a part of the mechanisms of government in the application of social order in the nineteenth century will be the theme which underlies the opening chapter.

But the construction of district nursing, health visiting, mental, school and industrial nursing also took place within other competing and parallel public discourses including those of eugenics, the management of poverty, national efficiency, imperialism and feminism.

Concerns, discourses and policies

The use of the term 'discourse' has proliferated in recent years and is in constant use throughout this section which places the construction, reconstruction and practices of community nursing within certain discourses and regimes. It is important therefore that a working definition of this crucial concept is clearly understood. Foucault's definition of power as diverse and embodied in practices, and not solely as a class-based economic structure, is an essential ingredient in an understanding of his use of discourse analysis and the concept of discursive regimes. A discourse is a construct of power and *knowledge*. In essence, he was concerned with the question, what is knowledge? How do we know what we believe to be 'the truth'? He believed that knowledge could be the subject of an archaeology whereby its roots could be uncovered as an ancient building could be uncovered and understood (Foucault 1974).

The theory of discourse is therefore an attempt to uncover the meaning of a body of knowledge. This is to accept that definitions of certain truths such as definitions and practices which centre on 'disease' or 'madness' have been constructed at specific historical times and junctures. So concepts such as 'disease' and 'madness' are not static, they are constantly in process of change. 'Madness' in the nineteenth century was a totally different construct, subjected to different practices and was a different 'truth' than the same category of 'madness' at the present time (Fox 1997). Nevertheless, both were products of a truth constructed in discourses that posited a knowledge which became the basis of medical and nursing practices.

A discourse makes a knowledge possible, it creates a system of rules, statements and practices which then mediates power to claim a 'truth' and make statements and eventually policies which claim to be based upon this speaking of the truth. There is, therefore, a relationship between power, knowledge and discourse. An analysis of discourse therefore studies the language through which a knowledge is carried and the sets of social relationships and practices which this connection constructs. Discourses therefore create a 'regime of the truth', this regime is linked to systems of power which constantly sustain, reproduce and extend it (Foucault 1980).

An example of this is given by Sarah Nettleton (1995) in her analysis of the development of dentistry in the nineteenth century. She pinpoints the discourse which created the 'truth' that there was a relationship between sugar and dental caries. Some texts supported this connection, others opposed it, but the debates and disagreements were all conducted within that regime of the 'truth'. David Armstrong (1986) argues a very similiar case for the 'invention' of infant mortality by medical statisticians in the latter decades of the nineteenth century. The reality was that high rates of infant mortality had always existed, but with more sophisticated calculations and techniques of diagnosing causation, a discourse of causes and the construction of it as a 'social problem' emerges as a truth. This 'truth' was then embodied in institutions, practices of medical science and health visiting, public health and education, and social policies. Everyday practices, publication of texts and pamphlets, regulations and policies all further amplify and construct the 'truth' of infant mortality as a social problem which could be solved by surveillance, regulation and administration.

In the first two chapters, we shall be using the concepts of discourse to study the emergence of various regimes of the 'truth' which informed practices and professional organisation of community nursing from the nineteenth century to the present day.

In the third chapter, we adopt a different perspective and focus on both the construction of different communities in Britain and the significance of the concept of 'community' for current social policies. It will be argued that, as in the nineteenth century, branches of community-based nursing especially health visitors and school nurses, are being utilised in the governmentality of a society experiencing social and economic change.

Finally, an analysis of current policies and a view from the 'front-line' of community nursing are presented. What are the experiences and meanings given to their social reality by community nurses themselves? What does it mean to be in the front-line today? We look at the *effect* of the 'truth' of policies and discourses based upon the management of poverty, the medicalisation of child surveillance, the 'ease' of day surgery, and the containment of mental illness. Community nursing is a construct, it is practised within certain 'regimes of the truth' which are now, as always, in process of change. It is concluded that the further challenge to community nurses will be to demonstrate that their nursing interventions span care, cure and control. They must also be able to show how their interventions can foster the image of a civilising profession which is intent on reforming and redirecting the lives of people who have been socially excluded from society.

CHAPTER 1

Public Health and Social Order: The Construction and Consolidation of Community Nursing before the NHS

Introduction

This chapter traces the function and practice of community nursing from the nineteenth century until the foundation of the postwar welfare state and creation of the National Health Service. The branches of community nursing that are focused upon in this period are those of district nursing, health visiting, school, industrial and mental health (asylum) nursing. The development of midwifery is only peripherally referred to but has been the subject of many histories and sociological studies (Donnison 1977, Oakley 1984, Hunt and Symonds 1995).

This development will be placed within the framework of three primary concerns that, it is argued, dominated political and health discourses during this period.

- Containment of epidemics and social order
- Pauperism and the management of poverty
- Control of quantity and quality of the population

These three spheres of articulated concerns must be seen as inter-connecting and crossing over many discourses at different periods of time. They cannot be seen in isolation, together they formed an overall 'regime of the truth' which informed and constructed the practices and perceived purpose of community nursing. At the same time, community-based practices themselves reinforced the discourses and reflected a 'truth'.

This period of time, covering barely a hundred years, experienced rapid social upheaval during which the certainties of the previous eras were disrupted. The First World War of 1914–18 marked a watershed between the nineteenth and the twentieth century. After the war, new beliefs and discourses were formulated which connected to those of the previous century

7

but also looked to new solutions based upon science, psychology and planning. Community nursing was constructed in the period before the war, and its practices and purposes both consolidated and changed in the interwar period.

The construction of community nursing was also surrounded by other influences, especially that of the gendered division of labour and a development of feminism. It also took place within a social and economic structure that changed from one of nineteenth-century imperialist arrogance and self belief to that of interwar despair and political radicalism.

The main argument to be followed is that the construction of community nursing must be seen as a part of the governmentality mechanism. This operated throughout this period to administer social order and impose a discipline upon society. The nature of the 'problems' of social order change over time, but the essential necessity for control and administration of order does not. Social order was just as essential, if differently defined, after 1918 as it was in the previous century.

Within the three main spheres of concerns, there can be seen historical changes in the object and theories of causation of problems. But the overall function of community nursing as being in the 'front-line' in the struggle for social order remains a constant.

The fear of epidemics and social disorder

The occurrence of epidemics and the fear they engendered concerning contagion serve as an almost perfect metaphor for the fear of social disorder. Epidemics seemed to be the illustration of the vulnerability of all when confronted with the infection of the few. In order to both contain epidemics and to then prevent them recurring, a new and powerful role for the state in public health legislation was projected.

The first cholera epidemic in Britain occurred between 1831 and 1832. It was initially concentrated in the port areas of London, Liverpool, Bristol and then spread to Exeter and Birmingham. Newman (1939) estimates that this first outbreak caused about 50,000 deaths in a population of approximately 23 million. But as these were concentrated in areas of population density, the effect was devastating. The panic and ensuing riots associated with cholera outbreaks posed a problem of social order. Some of the worst riots occurred in the slum areas where the inhabitants were the most vulnerable. This led to the association of disease and social unrest, it also led to the connection between disease and an 'outsider' or excluded class. The worst rioting took place in the Irish 'ghettoes' such as the Seven Dials area of London (Wohl 1983). The policy of swift burial and cremation of the dead was the cause of the riots, people were frightened of the prospect of premature burial in unconsecrated ground and there was a suspicion that bodies were being used for anatomy lessons in medical training.

Cholera reappeared at intervals throughout the early and mid nineteenth century; in 1848, a severe outbreak in 1854, and in 1865. As we shall see, the later outbreaks of cholera mirrored the expansion of public health legislation and the involvement of local authorities in the provision of district nursing.

Another epidemic that was associated with Irish immigration and the overcrowded conditions of the slums was typhus. This was also known as 'gaol fever' and 'Irish fever'. If typhus appeared to be a disease of the slums and the socially excluded, typhoid attacked all classes even reaching to the Royal family causing the death of Prince Albert in 1861 and the near death of his son the Prince of Wales in 1871. Due to the low standard of water supplies to all institutions including Royal residences and public schools, typhoid was feared by all.

Influenza was probably one of the major killers of the poor. Child mortality was high for scarlet fever, over 95 per cent of all cases were children. Later in the century, diphtheria was a cause of high child mortality due to contaminated milk supplies. The incidence of diphtheria rose in the latter years of the century due to the increased proximity of children in the new schools. After 1880, the introduction of the school register was made in order to attempt to control infection in schools by means of notification and the isolation of affected children.

Smallpox also caused social unrest, but ironically this was primarily targeted against the prevention of the disease – vaccination. An epidemic in 1837 to 1840 prompted the passing of the first legislative moves to bring in compulsory vaccination of children in 1853. But it was always unpopular with many of the poor who viewed it with great suspicion (Smith 1979, Wohl 1983). Another epidemic in 1871 centred in London, prompted the Smallpox Act, legislation that supported compulsory vaccination with fines and imprisonment.

But probably the greatest scourge was tuberculosis, the 'white plague'. This affected all classes but was most prevalent in overcrowded urban working-class slum areas. Some occupations, such as tailoring, especially in the overcrowded conditions in the garment 'sweatshops', were especially vulnerable. By 1900, it was the second most common cause of all deaths.

The panic which surrounded periodic acute epidemics, and the fear of the long-term chronic diseases of poverty, also translated into the fear of contagion and contamination of 'madness' and degeneracy. Carpenter (1980), has placed the definitions of madness and insanity which underpinned the drive to build asylums during the latter years of the nineteenth century as a response of governmentality and the need to control. The fear of contagion and contamination spread from epidemics to definitions of madness and degeneracy. As sewers were built to clear away filth and waste, so asylums were erected to house the human 'waste'. Sewers and drains were the guiding metaphors for those who depicted the deviants of this time. 'Foul wretches' and 'moral filth' lay heaped in 'stagnant pools' about the streets. When they moved they were seen to 'ooze' in a great 'tide' (Pearson 1977:164).

The fear of degeneracy and its connection to disease was evidenced by the passing of the Contagious Diseases Acts from 1864 onwards. Like connotations of madness, definitions of immorality and degeneracy were more easily applied to some groups than others, with women frequently seen as the carriers. The implementation of these Acts in garrison and port towns, was aimed at eradicating the spread of venereal disease in the army and navy. It involved the forcible medical inspection and incarceration of women defined as 'common prostitutes' and initiated a movement of opposition that brought together middle-class feminists and Trade Unionists in coalition against what was seen as the 'legal rape' of working-class women and girls (Walkowitz 1982). For many, this action on behalf of the state was a step too far in the imposition of social order and was opposed on both class and gender lines.

But the presence of epidemics as an inherent feature of everyday life caused a problem of social order. They robbed a society of a feeling of permanence and control of the future and in order to contain and prevent them recurring, measures had to be taken which would challenge other deeply held beliefs in the non-interventionist nature of the state.

Public health, social order and medicine

The beginning of the nineteenth century had seen a diversity of approaches to the protection of the population from diseases; from the 'medical policing' tactics of Germany to the 'voluntarist' free-market philosophy of Britain. Revolutionary France had initiated a system of state-based services including medical inspections, clinics, nationalisation of hospitals and community health inspectors (Porter 1999).

But the epidemics of cholera and other diseases that spread throughout Europe by the mid nineteenth century were to reveal the existing measures as ineffective.

'Cholera concentrated people's minds' (Porter 1999:409) and a variety of new discourses and solutions were presented. The existing system of quarantine was tried in order to combat the first epidemic in 1831 in Britain but it was not successful. In an era of 'free' trade, mobility of labour and the crowding together of people from many localities into slum areas, quarantine was no longer a feasible option.

Armstrong (1993), sees this as the last throw of the old system and the beginning of the 'golden age' of public health and sanitary reform. Quarantine was based upon the belief that diseases were geographically based, the movement of people was restricted as they were carriers of disease from place to place but disease itself was endemic to a specific site. The new discourse of sanitary reform was based upon the belief that sickness and poverty were inextricably and dangerously linked. A belief in sanitary reform within a newly industrialising society became merged with fears of pauperism and disorder which were illustrated by epidemics.

Reform of the Poor Law in 1834 under the increasing influence of the Benthamite Utilitarian philosophy of 'the greatest happiness for the greatest number' was the first move of the new sanitarian order (see Table 1.1). The figure of Edwin Chadwick dominates all histories of the imposition of the sanitarian and Utilitarian system of combating disease and poverty. Chadwick's original idea that by quarantining the feckless paupers in workhouses and deterring dependency upon the public purse, poverty itself could be eradicated, proved overly optimistic. Chadwick then moved to the premise that the causation of poverty was as much due to sickness as it was to fecklessness and this conviction underpinned the development of the science of epidemiology and public health legislation.

Table 1.1   Landmarks of state involvement in health and social welfare before 1945

1834	Poor Law Amendment Act – curtailed outdoor relief – set up workhouses, principle of less eligibility institutionalised
1848	Public Health Act – set up local boards of health in areas of high mortality
1872	Public Health Act – Sanitary authorities set up nationwide
1875	Public Health Act – enabled local authorities to set up hospitals, sewage collection and supply clean water out of rates
1890	Housing of the Working Classes Act – beginning of local authority provision of public housing
1904	Inter-Departmental Government Committee on Physical Deterioration set up to investigate state of the nation's health
1906	School Meals service for 'needy' children
1907	School Medical Service
1907	Registration of Births Act – enabled health visitors to monitor new births
1911	National Insurance Act – contributory, dependents not included, available to certain groups of workers earning less than £160 pa, paid sick pay, limited medical benefits. 90% of married women excluded
1918	Maternal and Child Welfare Act – development of health visiting, clinics set up by local authorities, home help service developed
1919	Addison Act – Local authorities given responsibility and subsidies to assess housing need and build houses
1924	Wheatley Act – increased state subsidies for public housing. Large council estates begin to develop
1929	Local Government Act – Local authorities take over old Poor Law infirmaries and Public assistance Committees replaced Boards of Guardians
1930	Greenwood Act – subsidies for programmes of slum clearance
1931	Means test introduced
1935	Publication of government report on increased rates of maternal mortality
1936	Agricultural workers included in National Insurance scheme
1938	Domestic servants included
1938	Barlow Commission – to set up national plan of housing development
1940	Emergency Medical Service – nationalisation of hospitals
1940	Evacuation of children from urban areas
1942	Beveridge Report published – blueprint for new welfare state

It is important to realise that in Britain the development of public health and the sanitary reform movement although led by Chadwick, a civil servant and involving many feats of civil engineering, also heralded the entry of the medical profession into public administration and governmentality. The first Poor Law Commission was set up in 1837 under Chadwick, and consisted of three doctors, Kay-Shuttleworth, Southwood Smith and Arnott, all of whom had an interest in epidemiology and the significance to health of the living conditions of the poor. The results of their researches into the conditions of the urban poor led to the imposition of public health legislation on water supplies, sewage disposal, pollution control, food adulteration and notification of diseases which were such a feature of Victorian Britain during the latter half of the century. The identification in 1854 of cholera as a water-borne disease by John Snow, a doctor working in the Soho district of London, was to be a further impetus to the sanitary reform movement. Snow himself was to become one of the leading figures in the sanitarian movement. The development of public health legislation within a bureaucratic state administration as the principle means of preventing epidemics was not without political opposition.

The overt state intervention that the sanitarian movement demanded was in direct opposition to the dominant philosophy of laissez-faire and an adherence to a 'voluntaristic' system of public health measures.

After the passing of the first Public Health Act in 1848, the growing involvement of local authorities in the regulation and control of pollution and 'offensive trades' went against the belief in 'free' trade and individual autonomy. *The Times* articulated the opposition of many of the middle-class rate payers and dominant interests when it proclaimed in 1853, 'We prefer to take our chance with cholera than be bullied into health' (cited in Porter 1999:412).

But the discourse of sanitary science was well established by the latter decades of the century. In some ways this discourse incorporated elements of the older one of 'miasma' theory with its focus upon the geographical location of disease. The concept of hygiene was now constructed and placed as a mediator between the external environment and the site of the individual human body. This shift illustrated, 'a new boundary which marked a separation from the space of the body from the space of geography' (Armstrong 1993:396).

Once this concept of hygiene had taken root, the public health legislation on clean water, sewage disposal and regulations on the burial of the dead, can be seen as a means of regulating the two-way transmission of polluting substances *between* the body and the environment. Much of this legislation depended upon the application of civil engineering rather than medical science. But the medical profession had staked its claim to direct this new relationship between individuals and the environment in the cause of prevention of epidemics. All the sanitary legislation that followed from the initial 1848 Act was directed by the newly created Medical Department of the Privy Council under the administration of John Simon. In reviewing the new role of the state in the prevention of diseases, Simon wrote,

> It has interfered between parent and child...between employer and employed...
> between vendor and purchaser...Its care for the treatment of disease has not been
> limited to treating at the public expense such sickness as may accompany destitution:
> it has provided that in any sort of epidemic emergency organised medical assistance,
> not peculiarly for paupers, may be required of local authorities.... (Simon 1868,
> quoted in Porter 1999:414)

But this new role required the personal one-to-one intervention of health care professionals. It was within this space, created by the separation of human bodies from their geographical location, that community nursing was first constructed.

Nursing and social order

If we approach the history of the foundation of nursing in the nineteenth century through the lens of the theory of governmentality, it is clear that nursing was placed 'in the front line in the techniques of pastoral government' (Nelson 1997). In the industrialising and uprooted society of the early nineteenth century, the practice of nursing took on a 'worldly' and secularised complexion. Histories of nursing (Abel-Smith 1960, Dolan 1973, Baly 1986, 1987), emphasise the drive in Protestant Britain to remove nursing from its Catholic connotations and into the realm of 'good works' and public duty: primarily performed by women. The figure of the woman as the bringer of civilisation fed into the sanitarian discourse based upon the bringing of order and discipline into the anarchy of industrialisation. The figure of the nurse was an essentially female construct. Except in the asylums and workhouse infirmaries where sex segregation meant the employment of males to attend to other males, the activity of nursing was seen as an extension of 'natural' female attributes. It was this ideological connection between nursing and innate feminine characteristics that was politically utilised by Nightingale and others to push for nursing reform (Holliday and Parker 1997). But, as Showalter (1981) points out, this was an essentially positive alternative to the destiny of wife and mother which was asserted (Showalter 1981:410).

Florence Nightingale, of course, exerted great influence over the direction of nursing practice in its initial stage of development. She was a firm believer in sanitarianism and gave as the four main causes of disease; agglomeration of sick under one roof, deficiency of space per bed, deficiency of fresh air, deficiency of light (Nightingale 1859). In this basing of causation of disease upon social-environmental conditions rather than on the individual medical model, Nightingale set out a specific path for nursing practice separate from medicine.

But the actual construction of nursing and the deployment of nurses was placed firmly within the mid nineteenth century structure of gender and class.

Histories of nursing (Dingwall et al. 1988) describe the many elements that surrounded the construction of the 'new model nurse': the influence of religion, enthusiasm for public health, and the demand by middle-class women for a useful occupation. Nursing was also caught in an identity crisis (which still exists). Was it to be a profession for educated ladies or a branch of domestic service? Abel-Smith (1960) has chronicled this social class dichotomy and its significance for recruitment throughout the late nineteenth and early twentieth century. But there was also a discernible division between what was seen as the ideal recruit for hospital nursing compared to community-based nursing. Home nursing was seen to require a higher calibre of recruit. 'The District Nurse must...be of a yet higher class and of a yet fuller training than a hospital nurse...the doctor has no one but her to report to him. She is his staff of clinical clerks, dressers and nurses' (Nightingale 1876, quoted in Baly 1986:128, Dingwall et al. 1988:178).

It was to this 'higher-class' community-based nursing that the everyday responsibility for the containment of epidemics and the implementation of social order was to be placed.

Containment and everyday management of social disorder

There were two routes through which the containment of epidemics and social order among the population on an everyday basis were to be achieved: institutionalisation of paupers and the mad, and home nursing and social visiting for the 'rescue' of the 'deserving' poor.

Under Poor Law legislation after 1834, the workhouse had been constructed as a site within which to contain the 'undeserving' poor, those who had failed to keep themselves from being a drain on the Parish funds. The Poor Law refused outdoor relief to the able-bodied, and this system of 'less eligibility' meant that conditions inside the workhouse must be seen to be harsher than those existing outside. The workhouse was not only, at the same time, a punishment for poverty and a deterrent from claiming benefits but also a place of last resort for the sick, disabled and insane. Within the organisation of parish relief, there was no distinction between the sick and the able-bodied, therefore, the infirmary became an indistinguishable part of the workhouse. Unmarried mothers made up a large proportion of the workhouse population and it was often their job to nurse other pauper women as an act of reparation for the 'help' they had received. The workhouse was used to effectively quarantine the paupers from society and therefore prevent an epidemic of poverty.

In the same way, definitions of madness were used to classify those whom, Carpenter (1980) argues, could not be a part of the new market economy and disciplined work ethic and whose irrational behaviour required control. Under the Lunatic Asylums Act of 1845, local authorities were required to build asylums to contain the insane (80 per cent of whom were paupers) in every locality. Prior to this date, many asylums operating under the ideal of the moral restraint of the insane and of the creation of a therapeutic community, already existed. Definitions of madness and degeneracy multiplied and by the closing decade of the nineteenth century the number and size of asylums and asylum populations had greatly increased (Showalter 1989, Scull 1996). The number of asylums in England and Wales increased from 24 in 1850 to 66 by 1890, and the average number of patients from 297 in 1850 to 802 by 1890 (Scull 1993:281). Carpenter (1980), describes them as 'custodial dumps' in that their purpose was 'to legitimate further the custodial warehousing of these, the most difficult and problematic elements of the disreputable poor' (Scull 1979:219).

It was to manage and control the inmates of these 'warehouses' that asylum nursing was constructed. From its inception, asylum nursing was dominated by working-class males who were called 'keepers' or 'attendants' rather than 'nurse' which denoted a female 'calling'. They were the equivalent of the 'handywoman' class in nursing (Dingwall et al. 1988). In many ways, the asylum was based upon the social structure of the manor house, with the administration in the hands of the gentry or professional class and the 'keepers' in the position of domestic servants or labourers (Digby 1985). The wages for both male and female keepers were low and based upon those of agricultural labourers in the surrounding area. Carpenter (1980), argues that the bad working conditions and long hours prompted the development of a Trade Unionism among the asylum workers who were seen as members of the 'dangerous classes' themselves. A contemporary account described them as:

> The unemployed of other professions... if they possess physical strength and a tolerable reputation for sobriety it is enough, and the latter quality is frequently disposed with. (Browne 1837, quoted in Mackintosh 1997:234)

But it was to these members of an underclass that the everyday management of the pauper and insane, the 'waste' of society, was entrusted.

In contrast, the nursing and education of the sick poor in their own homes was to be entrusted to a new type of nurse. The 'first administrative use of nursing to control epidemics' and to attend to the sick poor at home (Dean and Bolton 1980) occurred during the cholera epidemic of 1854 in Oxford. Nurses were engaged to visit the houses of the sick poor and paid for by the local Board of Guardians. The development of home nursing can be traced to many factors including religious sectarianism and the desire to achieve 'value for money' for the public purse. As records show, many saw it as a means of saving on the poor rate. Dr. Hurry, in 1898, described the district nursing service as 'value for money' in that it saved hospital expenses and returned the breadwinner to employment, thus rescuing a family from pauperism (Baly 1987:42).

The foundation of district nursing was particularly associated with the Quakers and the Anglican movement and had an emphasis on 'good works'.

But this was to carry its own set of contradictions, the nursing of the sick poor had been regarded as a Christian 'duty' but, with increasing state intervention in the form of local authority funding during the latter decades of the nineteenth century, this became seen as more of a 'right'. It was multicultural and multi-denominational Liverpool which was the centre for the initial construction of the service by William Rathbone, a Quaker who had converted to Unitarianism. Liverpool had, of course, a high rate of Irish immigration and was a city of great religious conflicts and divisions. Many of the early home nurses were primarily Bible missionaries who combined home nursing with evangelism.

Britain, in the nineteenth century, was not yet an urban society despite the emphasis on the living conditions of the new manufacturing towns by public health policies. The majority of the population still lived in rural areas and the need for both management and education of the agricultural poor was just as pressing. Interestingly, the foundation of a rural service had roots in Fabian socialism. The Mallesons, a Fabian couple in Gloucestershire were the first to raise funds for the setting up of a village-based nurse-midwifery service. These village nurses, recruited from and living among the villagers, were less qualified than the new model nurses. The existence in rural areas of the village nurse–midwife was to cause great intra-professional conflicts up until the founding of the NHS in 1948 (Fox 1993).

The growth of asylums during the second half of the century led to the construction of 'keepers' who were responsible for the containment of the mad but who also were seen as being of a dangerous nature themselves. At the same time, however, district nursing was constructed within a set of discourses concerning not just the containment of epidemics but also the management of poverty and the education of the poor for their own survival. Asylum nursing took place within the site of a public institution but one which was hidden from public scrutiny. District nursing took place in the private sphere of the home but was charged with a public duty – that of the administration of poverty and the prevention of pauperism.

The management of poverty

The discourses of the nineteenth century on poverty concerned its management, not its eradication. Poverty was seen as an essential component of the new Capitalist economy. As Chadwick himself stated 'banish poverty and you banish wealth'. It was pauperism that was defined as the essential evil to be destroyed (Dean and Bolton 1980). Political and ideological opposition to both state intervention and charitable support was based upon the view that it was the environment of poverty which caused moral and physical degeneracy. The poor needed to be educated and trained but not directly aided. Part of the training of the poor was concerned with imposing cleanliness and order upon their existence to prevent them from sliding into becoming a dangerous 'mob'. This, in differing strategies, was to be the role for district nurses and health visitors.

District nursing, often funded and managed by voluntary organisations, had a dual purpose; the nursing of the 'deserving' sick poor and the teaching of higher standards of hygiene and household order. Florence Nightingale saw the role of district nurse as that of nurse–teacher and guide to the poor:

> The district nurse has to show them their home clean for once; in other words, to do it herself, to sweep and dust away, to empty and wash out all the appalling dirt and foulness . . . Every home she has thus cleaned has always been kept so. This is her glory. She found it a pig-sty; she left it a tidy and airy room. (Nightingale 1876, quoted in Baly 1986)

This illustrates that for district nurses it was through their 'practice' that the teaching would take place and not through the imparting of 'theory', this was to be placed within the new occupation of health visiting.

As the nineteenth century progressed, the work of caring for the 'deserving' poor shifted from the sphere of private charity to the evolving state sector of health care. This shift to state responsibility for the poor set up many ideological contradictions, not least for some people working in this sphere. The books of Margaret Loane, a district nurse who worked in both the London area and surrounding rural districts in the early years of the twentieth century, represent an articulation of the issues faced by the new professional nurse. She placed the blame for the problems of the poor, including ill health, bad housing and malnutrition, firmly on their own ignorance and fecklessness. She herself worked for a non-sectarian voluntary agency and was an advocate of the new professional ethos represented by the Queens Institute. She elaborated upon this new role for district nursing which in many ways has a very contemporary feel:

> What is needed in the homes of the working class is not a respectable charwoman with a three months veneer of training but a highly skilled nurse, who strictly confining her personal service to the more difficult parts of her own profession, organises and directs the labour of the patients' friends. (Loane 1909:230)

The discourse of the management of poverty was one of the major forces behind the construction of home nursing. The role of the home nurse was seen as pivotal both in times of epidemic when the unregulated nature of the poor became dangerously apparent, and in 'peace time' when the training of the sick poor was required as a preventive measure. Despite this dual role, the identity of the district nurse was clear cut, her primary function was to nurse the sick, it was illness which caused her to be sent for. But the emphasis in the management and government of the poor working classes shifted to that of prevention and improvement. There were two other parallel discourses that became linked to the management of poverty, those of imperialism and motherhood. In the latter decades of the century, eugenic concerns over the quality and quantity of the population also combined to produce a demand for new occupations in governmentality.

Imperialism, motherhood and the population question

The discourses of imperialism and motherhood became linked to the management of poverty. The fundamental relationship between the family and the state underwent a process of change during the last decades of the century (Davin 1978). This new relationship involved ideas of responsible motherhood as the antidote to the publicly recorded high infant mortality rate, especially prevalent among the urban working classes. In conferences on the 'epidemic' of infant mortality in 1906, blame was not placed on the working or living conditions of the poor but squarely on the 'ignorance of mothers' (Davin 1978:50).

The Fabian Society presented its manifesto on National Efficiency in 1901. It was a significant document in that it clearly set out a programme of social reform based firmly on state control. Politically, the discourse of National Efficiency cut across party lines and attracted many intellectuals and business entrepreneurs to its meetings (Searle 1971). Efficiency in all spheres of social and economic life was the organising principle. This standard was to be achieved by experts who were guided by the ethic of public service to reform and rationalise the non-regulated nature of British society and its resulting social ills. This rejuvenated social organisation would be achieved by the application of scientific methodology and then Britain would be 'fit' in Darwinian terms, to take its place as a world leader. Thus the discourses of imperialism, social efficiency and motherhood became inextricably linked with a eugenicist drive to improve the 'quality' of the population.

The Fabian belief that the low standards of health, education and housing of the population could only be raised via total state action (Mackenzie 1979:291), slowly gained ground during the early twentieth century. The discourses of poverty management, imperialism, motherhood and National Efficiency can be seen to exist separately but to be in a dynamic relationship with each other. They coalesced into a developing framework of an alternative political ideology based upon the collectivist solution of state intervention and control that was to gain hegemony by the interwar years. Central to this belief was the eugenicist conviction that the standard of the population could be raised by scientific breeding, environmental reform and a 'new sense of citizenship' (Weeks 1981:195). Motherhood now became the focus of state intervention, especially for those working-class mothers who were deemed 'irresponsible'. The figure of the mother in this project became at the same time the *cause* of moral and physical degeneracy and its *solution*. But who was to educate and train women into this new national duty of motherhood?

'New work and a new profession for women'
(Nightingale quoted in CETHV 1977:12)

The histories of health visiting (Baly 1973, Dingwall 1977, Davin 1978, Davies 1988, Dingwall et al. 1988), all illustrate the steady 'gentrification' of health visiting from its inception in the last decades of the nineteenth century in Manchester. From its beginnings, this new profession was based upon a set of contradictions and illustrated dominant gender and class identities.

The origin of health visiting was within the sphere of public health, but as women, health visitors were consigned to work in the private sphere of the home with mothers and children. Men, on the other hand, were allocated the public sphere of inspection and environmental control of factories and shops. There is also evidence that the first health visitors were in fact local working-class women who led by example (Davies 1988). However, as state legislation grew with public concerns over the quality of the population, so health visiting became the province of the educated middle-class woman.

The state created this new profession. By the early years of the twentieth century there was evidence of a decline in the birth rate, Dingwall (1977) has shown that this was a basic concern of the report of the Interdepartmental Committee on Physical Deterioration in 1904. This decline fuelled a national concern over the survival and quality of the babies being born and gave the impetus for the state sponsorship of health visiting. The Notification of Births Act of 1907 enabled health visitors to call on all new born babies and the following year the London County Council (LCC) required that health visitors possess either a medical degree, midwifery certificate or nurse training. The job of the health visitor was to teach working-class mothers to better their children's chances of survival and so to construct responsible citizens. Health visiting combined the roles of health inspector, social worker and teacher. Although the nursing aspect was not evident, there was a perceptible connection with health and disease. Unlike district nursing, however, the development of health visiting was firmly set within the parameters of education and theory and, although a career for women, it was not as unambiguously a 'natural female' occupation as nursing. Dingwall (1982:340) suggests that the organisation of health visiting always 'represented a compromise between enforcement and libertarian values'.

Health visiting required the exercise of authority by a middle-class professional woman over working-class and uneducated women. This was not without its tensions and antagonisms, Smith (1979:117) argues that there was a great deal of resentment felt by many of the poor at this intrusion. On the other hand, projects like the School for Mothers set up by local boards of health were well received by many women in working-class areas (Davin 1978:38).

Health visiting and district nursing are the two most prominent occupations within community nursing which were constructed at this time within a set of discourses on poverty, motherhood, eugenics and National Efficiency. There were also two other branches of nursing which came into existence within this set of discourses; school and industrial nursing.

Schoolchildren and working women

The focus upon the health of children prompted by fears of a declining birth rate and the new emphasis on its 'future citizens', lay behind the construction of the school medical services (see Table 1.2). The siting of services of a doctor and nurse within schools was accompanied by wider public health measures that illustrated this new concern over physical 'fitness'. Much of this concern had been prompted by the revelations of the appalling state of health of the young recruits to the Boer War in 1900. Following from the revelation that of the 20,000 recruits only about 14,000 were judged as physically fit for service (in Manchester only 1200 were accepted out of 11,000), the concerns about National Efficiency had prompted social legislation. The medical inspections in schools and the emphasis on physical education (PE) in the curriculum was an example of this concern.

The teaching of PE and the priority given to games and drill was a feature of the school curriculum after the establishment of a Medical Branch of the Board of Education in 1907. The emphasis on physical training was seen as an 'antidote to physical deterioration' and would 'help Britain retain her national and commercial supremacy, inculcate citizenship and solve the question of home defence' (Shee 1903, quoted in Welshman 1996:32). Although there had been individual instances of local Nursing Associations appointing nurses to look after the health of children in school prior to the Education Act of 1870, it was not until 1890 that the London School Board appointed a medical officer for all elementary schools. This appointment was prompted mostly by fears of infection and epidemics to which the new schools, especially in overcrowded urban areas, were especially vulnerable.

In 1904, the report of the Inter-Departmental Committee on Physical Deterioration (which had also sponsored health visiting) recommended: a school meals service, training of girls in mother craft, physical training for boys (prompted by the Boer War inspections) and warned of the dangers of juvenile smoking. In 1907, school medical inspections became the responsibility of local authorities and in the following year the Board of Education instructed the appointment of school nurses to assist in inspections and to treat minor ailments in elementary schools.

The responsibility for the health and social care of schoolchildren shifted from the private sphere of the home to the public sphere of state surveillance and intervention (Webber 1998). The health and welfare of women, specifically mothers, was also to become the subject of public health attention.

Women workers, who were regarded largely as children, had been the focus of 'protective' employment legislation throughout the nineteenth century. They were now targeted for health service provision. As early as 1852, a 'lady visitor'

Table 1.2   State and school children 1870–1939

1870	Forster Act – system of elementary education to be provided from local rates and government grants. School Boards set up – on which women can become elected members
1890	London School Board appoints medical officer for elementary schools following outbreaks of infectious diseases in schools
1897	Cleansing of Person Act – school inspection of children for vermin
1902	Balfour Act – Local Education Authorities (LEAs) set up. Statutory duty to provide elementary education to all children until age of 14
1904	Report of Inter-Departmental Committee on Physical Deterioration recommends: school meals service, physical education and games for girls and boys, training in mothercraft and cookery (girls), warnings of dangers of juvenile smoking
1906	Education (Provision of Meals) Act allowed educational authorities to provide meals for destitute children
1907	Education (Administrative Provisions) Act – set up school medical service, school medical inspection responsibility of local authority and Medical Officer of Health. Curative services remained with private doctors
1908	Board of Education circular to local authorities – improvement of sanitation standards, appointment of school nurses to assist medical inspections and to treat minor ailments, supply of spectacles to children and establishment of school clinics. Physical education becomes part of school medical service and installed in curriculum
1913	Mental Deficiency Act – local authorities to provide special schooling for 'mental defectives' and 'epileptics' in area
1918	Fisher Act – extends duties of LEAs to provide medical inspections to all children in elementary and secondary schools
1919	Ministry of Health takes over duties of school health services
1919	School dental services provided in some areas
1920	Child Guidance Clinics set up – referral of children with 'behavioural problems' in school
1929	Report of the Mental Deficiency Committee – mental deficiency among school children increasing. Term of 'dull and backward' introduced
1931	Hadow Report recommended abolition of single schoolroom, site, space design and ventilation in schools become guidelines. Open air classes and playing fields recommended
1933	The Health of the School Child Report by School Medical Service – lays stress on nutritional standards, exercise, fresh air – as solutions to malnutrition. Also showed social variations in vermin inspections by nurses
1933	Children and Young Person's Act – children could be removed from families because of 'neglect' and transferred to institution or foster home
1934	Milk Act – government grant to Milk Marketing Board to make milk available in schools for halfpenny a small bottle
1938	Birmingham Education Committee School Medical Officer's Report – extensive malnutrition in schoolchildren – only 2% had 'excellent' and 10% 'sub-normal' rates of nutrition

had been employed by the Courtaulds factory in Essex, a large employer of women, to set up a nursery for employees' children. Women were also given time off for breastfeeding in the factory nursery. In 1878, the first industrial nurse was employed by Colman's factory in Norwich, another large female employer. She was a district nurse who worked as a 'link' worker between the factory and the homes of the employees (Charley 1954). The health of women at work was regarded as being of importance in so far as women had the identity of potential mothers of the imperial race. In 1893, the first women Factory Inspectors were appointed to oversee women's health in industry, but as Jones (1994) reports, they faced great opposition from male inspectors and only a handful were employed to cover a million and a half female workers. Increasingly, a whole debate on the appropriateness of married women working was conducted within a moral framework as well as focusing on the question of its effect on the health and well-being of children. The ideal of the wife and mother at home constructing a safe and welcoming domestic environment for the family was a very powerful image by the end of the nineteenth century. But, for the poor, this was an impossible attainment. Women worked in overcrowded sweatshops, took in washing, or more frequently did 'homework' in one-roomed slums shared by the whole family.

The connection between female employment and infant mortality was often made by campaigners. The infant mortality rate which had been high throughout the nineteenth century, declined by 33 per cent between 1867 and 1907 but only for children between one and five years, the death rate for babies under one year remained as high at the turn of the century as it had been in 1860. But the connection between this and mothers' employment was by no means straightforward or uncontroversial. There were three main reasons given for the undesirability of married women's paid work; it reduced childbearing capacity, prevented breastfeeding and 'was detrimental to the moral fibre of society' (Jones 1994:13). But not all campaigners agreed, many saw the extra money brought in as more beneficial to raising the living standards of the family. Dyhouse (1978), reports on a survey in Birmingham in 1909 that found babies had a better chance of surviving beyond their first birthday if their mothers worked. The main problem for women and children was that they continued to work in 'twilight' areas not covered by the Factory Acts. Legislation restricting their working hours did not apply to the vast majority of the poor who continued to work outside the official public gaze often in dangerous and unhealthy circumstances for subsistence wages.

Most child labour was unrestricted and commonplace, working-class children had interrupted schooling due to the use made of them in paid work or, in the case of girls, taking on the care of younger brothers and sisters (Davin 1996). Surveys on the lives of poor families illustrated the sheer grinding day-to-day poverty which especially affected the health of women and children (Pember Reeves 1913).

But as state intervention in the field of health insurance and access to service provision grew in the early years of the twentieth century, the main target was that of the male breadwinner. The health and well-being of women and children tended to be the concern of public health measures, the education system and intervention by community-based nursing. Male health needs, on the other hand, were to be the province of health insurance, Trade Union organisation and government policies. Men in skilled and relatively well-paid manual work, belonged to a Friendly Society which covered them for hospital or General Practitioner (GP) treatment, but very few women were covered by these arrangements, especially if they were not formally employed in their own right. The Workmens Compensation Act of 1897 was aimed almost solely at male workers who could claim for injuries sustained in employment regardless of negligence. Trade Unions also offered security to members in terms of access to a doctor or medicine and also to hospital treatment, but this again was an almost exclusively male privilege. Women and children as dependents were not covered by the National Health Insurance Act brought in by Lloyd George in 1911. Approximately 90 per cent of married women were excluded from this contributory scheme and so were excluded from access to a doctor or to hospital treatment that the NHI conferred, this situation remained until the founding of the National Health Service in 1948.

By the early years of the twentieth century, public concern and policies over the health of the population were framed by discourses that posited different destinies and roles for men and women. A developed Capitalist industrial economy required men to be productive in the creation of wealth and military service and women to be productive in the domestic servicing and creation of a fit and healthy population. Children were seen as a public responsibility of the state as well as a private responsibility of individual families. This reality marked a great cultural shift from the beginning of the nineteenth century with the main concern of public health being the containment of epidemics.

The private sphere of the family became the site for public intervention aimed at improving the survival rate of children and the quality of future citizens. Poverty had become a condition to be monitored and managed in order to prevent pauperism. Those who were excluded from any form of productive contribution by mental or physical disability or illness were warehoused in institutions and placed 'out of sight and out of mind'. Branches of community nursing had been constructed and organised to carry out the face-to-face management, education, surveillance and support of the 'deserving' poor and women and children. But the advent of war in 1914 and the conditions of the following years were to produce a different but connected set of discourses which the social organisation of community nursing addressed.

War and aftermath, new concerns and discourses

The 1914–18 war changed British society and culture in dramatic ways. The impact of war altered the lives of both men and women and instigated a set of discourses that dominated social policy in the interwar years.

After 1918, there was renewed concern over the 'quality' of the population and, following from the massive death toll of the war, pressure to increase the birth rate. The incidences of mental and physical disability that many of the survivors suffered was also to have an effect on attitudes and treatment of mental illness.

For women, the war opened new doors of emancipation and access to work culminating in the granting of the franchise to women over 30 in 1918.

Historians differ as to the lasting effect on women's lives that the war engendered but although some of the gains were reversed in the interwar years, none the less, as Marwick (1974) has argued, the war experience is crucial to an understanding of British society and culture between 1918 and 1939.

War also changed the relationship between men and women. The world of strict segregation of roles became less secure and the position of the male breadwinner was to decline with economic depression whilst 'the gains they (men) made in the political sphere were to be offset by those made by women' (Bourke 1996:14).

The spectre of the war haunted the interwar concerns and health policies and, coupled with a belief in a new type of society, underpinned the dominant discourses. The construction and organisation of branches of community-based nursing and health visiting was already in place by the outbreak of war but was to be subject to new directions in the interwar years. The three dominant discourses that had surrounded and prompted the construction of community nursing in the previous century still existed but were re-interpreted and in some ways re-articulated, to address new concerns.

The problem of epidemics and social order still remained. Although diseases such as cholera and typhoid had now been almost eradicated, there were others that prompted public health campaigns. There was also the problem of the 'war psychosis', the increase in mental illness of the 'fit' men who had survived the war and demanded different treatment than had previously existed.

The management of poverty and prevention of pauperism remained relevant despite growing affluence in some areas. By the early 1930s widespread depression and mass unemployment reinforced the bad living conditions in specific areas which had not improved over the past century.

The 'quality' and 'quantity' of the population remained a dominant discourse. The war had crystallised many of the fears of 'moral degeneracy' and eugenicist ideas were paramount in debates on the birth rate and on birth control.

But the post-1918 world was also to produce new beliefs and cultural frameworks and allied concerns which fed into these discourses and which consolidated and directed community nursing practice before 1939. The new discipline of human psychology was developed, firstly to address the mental breakdown of servicemen during and after the war, and then to be applied in a universal way to define individual motivations, behaviour and deviancy. The belief in science and 'scientific' methods permeated medical and nursing practice and this was coupled with a political adherence to the application of planning to both the economy and society. Planning and the organisation of society on rational efficient lines was one of the dominant discourses of this period. With this belief went the enthusiasm for state intervention and control over previously 'private' spheres of life including the family and sexual behaviour. The increased numbers of women working in both the professions and the new industries also prompted fears that women would no longer be willing to fulfil their role as mothers and the so-called 'woman problem' also entered into public discourse. This period was also one in which social and economic inequalities gained in political focus. The popularity of the cinema, the radio and the development of the popular press meant that the divisions in British society became visible. Socialism and Fascism both gained adherents, and ideas of a planned and national health service within an overarching welfare state gained currency. This cultural map included the existing discourses based upon social order and the improvement and control of the population. Community nursing was to play an important part in this postwar modernist world but firstly it was to be reorganised and professionalised.

As we shall see, the increase in the state organisation, funding and professionalisation of community nursing occurred within a set of discourses and ideologies which dominated the interwar years. Some of these had been in existence prior to the war, but others were a result of the great upheaval that war had brought to British society. One such change was the introduction of psychology and psychiatry to British culture which began to transform ideas about madness and its treatment, child development and social deviancy. This was also to have an impact on the practices of community-based and mental nursing.

Psychology and new forms of intervention

The experience of war was to challenge both the medical model of madness and distinct biological definitions of masculinity and femininity. For the first time the focus of psychiatry was upon men rather than women (Showalter 1989). As early as the winter of 1914, there were indications of a high percentage of mental breakdown among the wounded officers and men. This was to become a war-induced epidemic. By 1916, neurasthenia accounted for 40 per cent of casualties in combat, and by 1917, it was reported that 20 per cent of discharges were on the grounds of 'neurosis' (Bourke 1996:109). By the end of the war, 80,000 cases had passed through the army medical service that had created an enormous strain on existing facilities. New hospitals had to be constructed as the old institutions could not cope with the demand.

In the beginning, 'shell shock', as it came to be popularly called, was treated with disbelief by the medical establishment and the sufferers were defined as cowards or 'malingerers'. But this could not be sustained as the effects were felt by more and more men. Importantly, these were men who were defined as physically fit and in fact were popularly thought of as heroes. In recent years many women writers (Showalter 1989, Bourke 1996), have defined this as a 'crisis of masculinity' when definitions of male behaviour became uprooted. Interestingly, social class definitions of the nature of the mental illness also proliferated; the officer class were diagnosed as suffering from 'neurasthenia' and the men were diagnosed as suffering from 'hysteria' a term previously reserved solely to diagnose women (Showalter 1989:175).

The epidemic of mental breakdown also forced a change upon the medical establishment. The theories of Freud and psychiatric techniques including early versions of electroconvulsive therapy (ECT) were applied in treatments. The belief that a psychiatric or emotional disorder was possible even among the physically able and fit served to divide body and mind in medical diagnosis and treatment. This was to have a far-ranging impact on other areas of social life including child development and industrial relations.

In terms of social policy, the effects were also significant. In 1920, the War Office convened a committee of inquiry into the incidences of neurasthenia and by 1921 there were over 65,000 men receiving pensions for mental disability. Even by the 1930s, 36 per cent of ex-servicemen in receipt of a war pension were listed as 'psychiatric casualties' (Bourke 1996:109).

The 'masculinisation' of mental illness also had significance for mental nursing. Although, as we have seen, asylum nursing from its inception included high numbers of men, due to the now high numbers of male patients the occupation itself took on a masculine approach to professionalisation.

The predominantly male attendants in asylums had, before the war, begun to unionise. They formed the National Asylum Workers Union in 1910 and affiliated to the Labour Party in 1914 and to the TUC in 1923. The bargaining strength of the union became apparent when it achieved in 1920, a shorter working week, a guaranteed weekly wage and equal pay for men and women (Carpenter 1980:143).

This identification with a skilled trade rather than a 'vocation' also affected the position of mental nursing registration in 1919. There was to be an almost constant battle during the interwar years over registration between the Medico-Psychological Association (MPA) and the General Nursing Council (GNC) over the control of certification (Dingwall et al. 1988:132). The MPA certificate was desired by the bulk of the nurses as it carried the status of a 'medical' rather than a 'nursing' identity, and was of course a masculine rather than a feminine definition. The membership also feared that the gains made by them through unionisation would be undermined by a flood of cheaper female labour in the service. But the financial and economic crisis which followed the war meant that, despite the increase in the patient population and in developing techniques of psychiatry, unemployment in mental nursing and wage cuts depressed the occupation.

The Mental Treatment Act of 1930, promised much but in the midst of the economic depression may have accomplished little. The separation of mental hospitals and the Poor Law under the Act meant that mental illness was no longer officially associated with pauperism and the definitions of 'idiot', 'lunatic' and 'asylum' were abolished. There was an emphasis on preventive consultation and treatment and on voluntary admission. Nevertheless histories of the period conclude that mental nursing remained a 'humble occupation' (Dingwall et al. 1988:135) and the public perception of mental health services was not much altered. But the influence of the science of psychology as an explanation of individual and social behaviour was to have great significance to new models of social organisation and welfare. As we shall see, the professionalisation and reorganisation of other branches of community nursing was also affected by ideas of science and rationality and practice was to reflect the impact of the new science of psychology.

Health policies, the state and professional nursing

The war had two main effects on the organisation of health care to the public; the setting up of a distinct government Ministry of Health in 1919, and the state professionalisation of nursing. The death toll of the war also reinforced the movement for infant welfare that had begun in the latter years of the nineteenth century. Children's survival and development became even more of an important issue as the losses of the war mounted. As one contemporary writer expressed it, 'father had been torn apart by shrapnel or smothered by poison gas, his small sons and daughters, the parents of the future took the spotlight as the hope of the nation' (Baker, quoted in Bourke 1996:17). A Ministry of Health was set up in 1919 under Dr Addison, and a report on the reorganisation of the health services was commissioned. In this report by Lord Dawson (a famous physician) published in 1920, which was 'ahead of its time' (Baly 1973:143) an embryo national health service was proposed. It recommended the state organisation of medical services based upon district hospitals and primary care centres staffed by GPs. But the financial crisis which followed the war meant that this ambitious programme was to be shelved until the advent of the Second World War. There was, however, one significant policy change enacted in the depression years. In 1929, the organisation of Poor Law hospitals was taken over by public health departments of local authorities. In many areas, this led to an expansion of the hospital service as well as an effort to rid the hospitals of their stigmatising image.

The First World War turned the spotlight on nursing as a worthwhile and desirable job for a woman. Although this positive image had to some extent been a product of wartime propaganda with images of 'angels' comforting wounded heroes, nevertheless, nursing had gained a high profile by 1918. The social composition of nursing had also undergone a change: 'by 1917, there 45,000 women doing nursing and a number of these were middle-class girls doing hard and rewarding work for the first time' (Baly 1973:142). In 1919, after 50 years of dissension and argument between the pro and anti factions to registration and qualification by examination, the Nurses Registration Bill was passed. For the first time, men were included and there was a separate section for mental nursing. In 1925, the first state examinations were initiated and these were the only qualifications of professional acceptability.

Community-based nursing unlike hospital nursing, was undertaken in the private sphere and often operated in a less visible and informal way and was therefore more difficult to regulate. In rural areas especially, the distinction between district nursing, health visiting and midwifery was often non-existent, with one person being enabled to undertake all three specialisms. This was especially common practice in sparsely populated rural areas. Although there was a positive side to this integrated working, 'one woman in one area formed a closely integrated service to a common end, and the woman who provided this service was guide, philosopher and friend to a whole neighbourhood' (Stocks 1960:160).

Nevertheless, it must also be remembered that the nurse was not paid separately for each specialism, work on the rural district therefore was often relatively badly paid.

District nursing remained organisationally fragmented throughout the inter-war years until the coming of the National Health Service in 1948. District nursing associations were the agencies that provided nursing services before 1948, they employed nurses and were locally based, often with voluntary committees responsible for funding. They also worked in conjunction with The Queens Institute that had been founded in 1887 for the training of district nurses, and qualification as a Queens nurse carried with it a mark of high status and relatively high pay. But as Fox (1993) records, in rural areas there was often confusion by local authorities who preferred to employ local 'village nurse–midwives' rather than the more prestigious and expensive Queens nurse. But by the mid 1930s, with increasing state regulation, in order to gain county council affiliation, local committees had to employ Queens nurses as superintendents in all areas. This was one example of the occupational tensions and intra-professional rivalry which was evolving following the state professionalisation process. But the organisation of district nursing via local associations was by the 1930s only kept in existence by the injection of funding by local authorities, and this was bringing it closer to a state service (Stocks 1960).

Health visiting, on the other hand, became more clearly professionalised and moved to the centre of state policies with the new focus on child welfare. Pressures for qualification grew and in 1916 the Board of Health recommended that health visitors should have both a sanitary inspectors and a midwifery certificate. In 1925, the health visitors certificate, awarded by the Royal Sanitary Institute, could be gained by a qualified nurse after six months post-basic training. By 1928, the employment of unqualified health visitors was prohibited, initially by the LCC and then more generally.

The state professionalisation process was fuelled by the Maternal and Child Welfare Act of 1918. This required local authorities to set up clinics and services to monitor the health of nursing and expectant mothers and children under five. This was to have a significant effect on health visiting. By 1918, the numbers of health visitors employed by local authorities had quadrupled (Dwork 1986). The work of health visitors expanded to include the investigations of stillbirths, tuberculosis control visiting, and moved to a universal service which included visits to middle-class and affluent families (Lewis 1980).

The discourse of science and planning surrounded much of this expanded role and influenced health visiting practice. The application of scientific methodology to childrearing was to be an important trend of the 1930s, especially among the middle classes. But there remained an outstanding problem to be confronted, the persistence of relatively high rates of maternal mortality.

Save the mothers

By the 1930s, the discourse on the quantity and quality of the population focused upon two main issues; the seeming reluctance of sections of the population to reproduce, and the enactment of public policies on improving the health of women and children.

The birth rate in Britain had declined faster than any other similar European country, it had fallen from 23.6 (per thousand) in 1901–05, to 19.9 in 1921–25, and in 1931–35 it was 15.0 per thousand. The picture was made even more alarming in the eyes of eugenicists by the fact that the marriage rate had in fact risen during this time. It was obvious therefore that many married women were refusing to become mothers. Who were the 'missing mothers'? The birth rate among the upper and middle classes had already declined by 1914, and a social class gradient in family size was an obvious element of fertility patterns. What was different in the interwar years was the spread of smaller families throughout sections of the working class. The birth rate among the skilled manual working class was virtually halved between 1901 and 1931, and by 1930 the average family size for this group of the population was 2.5 children.

The low birth rate and the declining infant mortality rate was however, counteracted by the relatively high rates of maternal mortality. Avoidable deaths from childbirth, the 'deep and continuous stream of mortality' (MoH 1937:51) had been the subject of governmental investigation since 1924. But the figures for maternal mortality for 1933 showed a rise of 22 per cent from 1923. The real significance of these figures when published in 1933 lay in their use within a discourse on 'safety' in childbirth. This was to be one of the most important political and public health campaigns of the interwar years. Histories of this campaign focus upon its organisational effects: increased hospitalisation of childbirth, the state organisation and employment of midwives in 1936, the development of obstetrics as a hospital-based discipline resulting in the 'male take over' of childbirth itself (Donnison 1977, Lewis 1980, Oakley 1986, Leap and Hunter 1993, Hunt and Symonds 1995). The discourse of 'safety' in childbirth carried two important issues; the advocacy of hospital as the safest site, a proposal which has been strongly refuted by Tew (1995), and the image of childbirth as a scientific and technological and public process far removed from pain, fear and potential death. Both of these components had an impact upon the popular perceptions of childbirth and maternity care. The official government-backed campaign for 'safe' childbirth stressed the necessity for the training of doctors and nurses, the development of new technologies, use of drugs and pain relief and the medicalisation and hospitalisation of childbirth.

But there was another view which gathered support in its explanation for the reluctance of women to become mothers. There was a popular belief, which entered into official publications, that modern women had perhaps become too 'soft' and 'civilised' for the rigours of childbirth and motherhood.

The report on the causes of maternal mortality published in 1937, contained the following astounding critique of the 'modern woman';

> The sensationalism of the popular press, the emotional stimulus of the films, the never ceasing impact of the radio, the speed of machines in factories and of the traffic on the streets, to which the physical reactions of men and women must be adjusted in this mechanical age, inevitably give rise to increased nervous tension. The fashion of slimming and the habit of cigarette smoking on the part of women are also features of the present age. (MoH 1937:117)

In one sense, this view recognised that women had changed in their lifestyles and expectations and that if the pro-natalist policies were to be achieved, the 'traditional' aspects of childbirth had to be eradicated. Childbirth had to become more scientific, streamlined and 'modern'.

Hospitalisation grew rapidly during the 1930s and was increasingly demanded by women themselves, mainly because hospital, under the supervision of a consultant obstetrician, offered access to the new technologies of pain relief (Hunt and Symonds 1995). Local authorities, notably the LCC, sought to make political capital out of provision of 'safe' childbirth and opened maternity units in the old Poor Law hospitals that had been passed to their control in 1929. Many of these units were newly built and often reflected 'state of the art' birth technology under the supervision of the increasing number of obstetricians. The increased use of antibiotics and sulphonamide drastically reduced the dangers of sepsis and was certainly the most important factor in the decrease in maternal mortality that began in 1937.

Although midwifery was the occupation to be most obviously affected by the drive for hospitalisation, with the 1936 Midwives Act effectively making them employees of the state, nevertheless, other branches of community-based nursing were also affected. The delineation between midwifery, district nursing and health visiting was broken as more and more midwives now practised within the hospital site. The ambiguities of nursing 'on the district' began to clear, and the object of individual occupational practices became more clearly defined.

For health visitors, the purpose and object of their practice, the education of working-class mothers, was being widened to include the middle class and was also to be affected by the shift towards the application of science to previously traditional and 'natural' tasks.

Scientific mothercraft

The belief in 'science' as both a philosophy and a method to be applied to the problems of society was one of the ideological features of the postwar era. The aims of health visiting of the Edwardian era, to 'educate' poor mothers into hygiene and nutrition, were now replaced by the belief in the scientific rearing of children to produce certain characteristics.

Motherhood and childrearing became a technical 'skill' underpinned by scientific theories and manuals on childrearing and child development proliferated, most of them written by male 'experts'. One of the most influential was Dr Frederick Truby King, whose theories on scientific and strictly programmed methods of feeding and child care, and even the showing of affection, influenced health visitor practice. But as Richardson (1993) points out, this strict scheduling of tasks probably had more influence on the middle classes than on the impoverished and overcrowded poor family. Nevertheless, this scientific approach altered the role of motherhood and childhood by focusing upon a developmental process that could be monitored and controlled by health visitors. There existed, however, a divide between theory and practice in this new movement. The theories gained adherence among predominantly male medical and psychiatric professionals but it was the female occupation of health visiting which had the responsibility of putting these ideas into practice. This often meant that health visitors were placed in the position of challenging traditional and popular methods of mothering.

One such challenge which health visiting practice engaged, was the opposition to dummies. As Gale and Martyn (1995) argue, the campaign waged by health visitors and childcare experts against dummy use (which halved between 1911 and 1930) was conducted on two levels. The 'unhygienic' nature of dummy use had always been attacked by health visitors but now it was opposed because it indulged 'babies' desires for comfort and pleasure and would be detrimental to their characters' (Gale and Martyn 1995:231).

The influence of behaviourist psychology was noticeable in the childrearing manuals and in popular magazines, as Ehrenreich and English describe, these ideas were part of a eugenicist drive to construct future citizens:

> Methods existed or were about to be discovered, in modern psychological laboratories for instilling workers with obedience, punctuality and good citizenship while they were still in the cradle and long before they had ever heard of trade unions or socialism. (Ehrenreich and English 1979:187)

Child Guidance clinics also made an appearance during the 1920s and 1930s, these were set up to deal with behavioural problems manifested at school. So that, as well as being concerned with physical development, the school medical service encompassed emotional and mental development. This was an illustration of the growing application of science to child development.

The well baby clinics that were held by health visitors in community clinics following from the 1918 Act also attracted opposition from the medical profession for their 'unscientific' nature. The clinics look 'homely' said a report, but 'are semi-social and unscientific' (quoted in Stacey and Davies 1983:34). But many GPs had cause to fear the impact of community clinics as many people used them in preference to paying a doctor's fee (Lewis 1986:22).

The shifts in both the management of childbirth and of childrearing towards a planned, scientific and medically-dominated approach were also reflected in other areas of social life.

Producing healthy children and workers

Once the nation's children were encompassed within the education system after 1870, the state's responsibility for children's health became central to education policies. What Mayall (1996:25) has called 'the politics of child health' during the interwar years were based upon the belief in a healthy programme of exercise, nutrition and fresh air. If individual mothers could be blamed for the bad health of their own children, then schools sought to counteract this by the universal application of physical exercise, open air classes and nutritional supplements.

The Edwardian emphasis on feeding pauper children, which was a foundation of the 1906 Education (Provision of Meals) Act, gave way to an emphasis on physical fitness and competitive games. It is essential to place this focus upon sport and physical education within the context of the considerable publicity given to sport by the totalitarian regimes of Nazi Germany and the Soviet Union during this period.

The health lessons learned in school, such as good table manners, a nutritional diet, rest, fresh air and exercise were to be taken home by children and act as an example to ignorant mothers. Physical, intellectual and social development were linked together in education policies which sought to bypass family and economic conditions and make children products of the system.

The Hadow Report of 1931, recommended the abolition of the single room primary school, the use of open air classes and physical recreation as well as guidelines on ventilation and space in schools. In 1937, the provision of open air spaces and playing fields was a part of the Physical Training and Recreation Act. Despite this movement of healthy schools, the responsibility for the health of school children remained a responsibility of the Ministry of Health and was not transferred to education until after the war in 1944.

The state and local authorities began to take more responsibility for the diet of children and pregnant women through the Infant Welfare clinics movement that gathered support from many quarters, including women's groups. Since 1922, local authorities had issued free and cheap milk to families with young children on a means-tested basis. Some areas also instituted a 'sunshine clinic' where 'rickety children and poorly fed mothers' (Lewis 1980:173), were given sunlamp treatment to correct dietary inadequacies. Under the Milk Act of 1934, a government grant was given to the Milk Marketing Board to make milk available to all children in schools at a minimum cost. This was only partially successful and by 1936 only 45 per cent of children were participating (Lewis 1980:187).

The belief that physical exercise was bad for women in that it made them sterile, unfeminine and unfit for motherhood, soon fell out of fashion by the interwar years (Jones 1994:70). Girls as well as boys were subjected to compulsory games in schools and physical fitness for women began to be actively promoted. The Women's League of Health and Beauty founded in

1930, was universally popular and 'keep fit' became a widespread craze. The emphasis on physical fitness for women, however, was influenced by the eugenicist desire to promote healthy motherhood, and was linked to the 'safe motherhood' campaigns. This interest in women's health was also apparent in workplace policies. If 'science' was being applied to the 'natural' female activity of childrearing then the opposite was happening in the new developments in welfare work in industry.

There, it was argued, the 'human factor' in monotonous industrial work must be recognised, analysed and encompassed by industrial nurses and welfare workers. This concern was prompted by the influx of large numbers of young women into heavy industrial production during the war. The health of women munitions workers especially had given rise to political concern. The formation of the Welfare Workers Institute in 1919, was an important step in the professionalisation of this branch of welfare and nursing work. The new directions were aimed at improving and monitoring the health and lifestyles of female workers. But this concern must be set against the reality of low wages for women and, even by 1939, the average wage for a single female was 30 shillings a week with the accepted 'poverty line' being 30s 9d. (Baly 1973:159). Nevertheless, women workers were to be the subject of many research studies into human relations in industry between the wars, most notable being the Hawthorne Studies in the USA.

After the First World War, many women engaged in heavy industry left their jobs (sometimes by coercion) and 'returned to the home' or domestic service. But a number of nurses remained in industry. In 1934, specialist training was recommended by the College of Nursing for qualification as an industrial nurse and this consisted of a specific programme within the six months' health visitor certification.

As well as the provision of formal health services, industry was also being affected by public health legislation and social policies that sought to modernise and improve working conditions. By the 1930s, the expansion of new industries employing mainly women and younger workers, and largely based in the South of England and the Midlands, brought new standards to industrial working conditions. Many of these well-organised firms offered their workers a range of welfare services including subsidised canteens, well-ventilated and lit areas, as well as leisure facilities and holidays with pay. Health measures such as mass screening for tuberculosis and the services of an occupational nurse were also put in place. New scientific production methods were accompanied by the provision of planned and regulated working environments. Although still in a minority, these new industries offered the benefits of a welfare state in miniature. The reality for many of the working class, however, especially in the depressed areas, was a life dominated by poverty, malnutrition and unemployment. The correlation between health and poverty formed a familiar but transformed discourse in the uneven economic and social change taking place.

Poverty and health

By the 1930s, the familiar discourse centring on the causation of poverty and its relationship to health, had entered a new phase. Increased monitoring and data collection by a range of bodies including the Medical Research Council, local public health officials, local authorities and the Medical Branch of the Board of Education, meant that a wealth of statistical evidence on the nation's health, was available to the public. But as Webster (1982) argues, this mass of evidence was also the subject of political divisions in interpretation. The official view of the government bodies was an 'optimistic' one, stressing the improvements in health that had been obtained since the end of the war. But the opposite view taken by many individuals who were broadly placed on the political left, was the 'pessimistic' one of a stagnation or even a deterioration in the health and living standards of the working class, especially in the areas of high deprivation and unemployment. This divide in interpretation called into question the neutrality and objectivity of the scientific status of 'facts'.

According to the official view, the incidence of malnutrition, for example, had by 1932 been virtually extinguished with only a recorded 1 per cent of the school population 'requiring treatment', compared to the figure of 15–20 per cent prior to the war (Webster 1982:112). But this was not a conclusion reached by many local medical officers of health. There was of course the problem of different methods of diagnosis, many of the methods used by school doctors were impressionistic and varied widely from area to area. A report published in 1935 (Betenson 1935, cited in Webster 1982:119), showed that diagnosis of malnutrition varied considerably between male and female observers, with women recording nearly six times as many incidences among the same group of children. McGonigle, a well-known public health doctor working in Stockton, published a much higher figure of 2.2 per cent of school children of the area suffering from malnutrition and a staggering 18.7 per cent suffering from 'subnormal nutrition'. His figures also showed 8 per cent of mothers suffering from malnutrition and 26 per cent suffering from subnormal nutrition (McGonigle and Kirby 1936:146).

The science of nutrition was now calculating the calorific value of foods and official guidelines were set out as to the protein and vitamin requirement of children and adults. Undoubtedly the diets of the unemployed were worse than those in work, in 1936 the nutritionist John Boyd Orr claimed that over 50 per cent of the population had insufficient real income to allow them to purchase the basic minimum of their nutritional needs (Boyd Orr 1936). The powerlessness of dieticians and others to intervene effectively to improve the health of the poor was obvious, 'The dietician can advise as to dietary but cannot supply the wherewithal to purchase the quantity and quality of foodstuffs recommended' (McGonigle and Kirby 1936:179).

This of course, was the real heart of the political division over the meaning of health statistics, the causation of poverty and resulting ill health could not be tackled primarily by medical advances or by the health services it could only come from the radical reorganisation of society and the implementation of a welfare state which provided a basic minimum income.

The evidence that poverty and its concommitants of bad housing, overcrowding, large families and inadequate diets was a primary cause of tuberculosis, dental decay, eyesight problems, anaemia, infection, and long term morbidity was overwhelming (Hutt 1933, McGonigle and Kirby 1936, Gloyne 1944, Webster 1982, Jones 1994), but consistently underplayed by the official accounts.

One reason for this blinkered approach was the fact that for some sections of the population health had improved but, as Webster argues, it was the differential between the more affluent and the deprived areas that was striking even allowing for an overall *average* improvement in some areas. All indices of health were calculated according to an average with very little notice paid to social class gradations. Likewise improvements in mortality rates can be shown to have slowed down under the impact of widespread depression. For instance the infant mortality rate fell from 83 (per 1000) in 1921 to 66 in 1931, 60 in 1941 and by 1946 to 43.

Maternal mortality, as we have seen, was one of the greatest public health issues, and official reports were anxious to deny the significance of social and economic factors. The report of 1937 had presented evidence to illustrate that 'women of the poorer classes do not run a greater risk in childbearing than those in comfortable circumstances' (MoH 1937:121). The class differential was hard to 'prove' by statistics alone, but many commentators remained far from convinced and newspaper reports of conditions in the depressed areas gave a vastly different picture (Hunt and Symonds 1995:107). The highlighting of black spots of maternal mortality led to the piloting of local schemes of provision of ante- and post-natal services. The Rochdale and Rhondda experiments are an illustration of local schemes which involved local authority-employed midwives, nursing and medical services, and the setting up of clinics. In 1936, the government approved a scheme to provide mothers in the Rhondda (the highest rate of maternal mortality) with free milk and this was later extended to the town of Jarrow under the Special Areas scheme (Lewis 1980:187).

Despite these limited schemes, however, there was an official reluctance to perceive of poverty as a primary cause of ill health and a shying away from the inevitable conclusion that a 'cure' for national ill health would require far more state intervention than the giving of individualistic health education or treatment.

Construction and consolidation of community nursing

This chapter began by setting out the dominating discourses that, from the middle of the nineteenth century to the eve of the war in 1939, were to surround and inform the construction of community nursing. Not only had community nursing been constructed in these years but also the practice had been professionalised and expanded. Yet this was a rather uneven development, some branches had advanced more than others but all had been framed by the discourses and public concerns which criss-crossed political and public debate.

The fear of epidemics that dominated the early part of the period had subsided by the twentieth century, but other fears had taken its place. Cholera and typhoid may have been eradicated but tuberculosis was still a major killer and the warehousing of the 'mentally unfit' still continued. Social order remained volatile and the existence of the poor threatened to engulf any major social advancements.

The management of poverty that was an essential ingredient of both district nursing and health visiting practice in the early stages of their development, had become a part of the organisational responsibility of the state and local government.

The organisation and funding of district nursing was fragmented between local voluntary agencies, local authorities and private concerns. But, by the 1930s, the figure of the district nurse was a familiar one and in many areas she was the representation of a public health service 'on the district'. This may be a rather romanticised description but it does convey the universal and widespread acceptance which district nursing had achieved.

The same could not really be claimed for health visiting. This was always a more ambiguous occupation than district nursing. Based on interventionist education rather than caring, health visitors were frequently the recipients of opposition and antagonism from the working-class population they were constructed to 'improve' (Lewis 1980:105). This was an occupation that was intrinsically connected to the eugenicist discourse based on the perceived decline of the quality and quantity of the population. This discourse gathered momentum after the First World War and allied concerns over the effects of poverty, ignorance and the belief in the scientific approach to childrearing consolidated the practice and viability of health visiting. But despite a higher profile and a more universal application for health visiting, the numbers being trained actually fell in the 1930s. One reason for this was that by then it had become a part of nursing and cuts in welfare services meant that many of those trained took up employment back in the hospitals.

School nursing had become established during the interwar years. The postwar emphasis on infant and child welfare meant that health education, medical inspections and surveillance entered into the school curriculum. Child health was one area in which state intervention had increased in the years from 1906 to 1939. Industrial nursing too had gained recognition. The increase of women into the industrial and commercial workforce both during and after the war meant that the welfare of female workers, especially, also became an interest of government. This interest was also fuelled by eugenicist ideals, but general concern over the future health of nation also meant that the health of male workers too was being more closely monitored by government and the trade union movement. As Bevin, then General Secretary of the Transport and General Workers Union, wrote in 1934,

> A tremendous contribution can be made to the health and happiness of a nation by placing at the disposal of productive industry an understanding branch of the medical and nursing profession thereby securing the health of the workpeople. (Charley 1954:107)

It is interesting to note that it is assumed here that the nurses would be 'understanding' and sympathetic towards the workpeople. Community nursing in most aspects was closer to the people both geographically and sometimes socially. Health visiting was an exception, as the demand for qualifications grew a more middle-class recruit began to enter. The nature of the practice of health visiting too meant that it took on a more directive and authoritarian aspect. But in the case of mental nursing, this remained not only a male-dominated job but also one that was overtly working class in organisation and political affiliation. Mental nursing had to some extent come out of the shadows by the interwar years with the increase and change of composition of the patient population, but it still was tainted with the stigma which adhered to mental health in general. But, at the same time, psychology had made an impact on the mental health services as well as on other practices.

All branches of community nursing had been constructed and had their practice consolidated within a framework of discourses and concerns over health, welfare and the social order.

Towards a new model of society

By 1939, Britain was a very different society from the one that had gone to war in 1914. The interwar years had produced many changes but had also seen the continuation of many of the problems and concerns of the nineteenth century. It was a period of great contradiction and diversity. The First World War had produced a cultural change, the certainties of the pre war world were shattered and new solutions for old problems were being sought. The political structure had also altered, the growth of the Labour Party and ideas of social equality and wider democracy entered into public debate. The influence of science and psychology meant that a new format was being sought for the provision of services. The health of the population became a central concern of government. Ideas for a state health service were already in the air and public health campaigns, as we have seen, centred more on the active promotion of health and fitness rather than protection from disease.

During the 1920s and 1930s the work and influence of public health departments had grown. Between 1919 and 1939 'some twenty pieces of legislation benefiting local health authority services were passed' (Lewis 1986:11). The focus of these departments had been largely on setting up health centres and implementing school services but they were also heavily involved in the administration of local municipal hospitals after 1929. Throughout this period, however, a division had grown between GPs and public health departments with the British Medical Association (BMA) often accusing public health of 'encroaching' on independent practices. Lewis (1986), argues that in fact many Medical Officers of Health were too focused upon clinical medicine and ignored their preventive role. There were, however, a minority of Medical Officers of Health who became very involved with debates on the social and economic factors of disease and believed that a future state service would enable them to put a type of 'social medicine' into practice.

Although women and children still remained largely outside of the state insurance schemes, nevertheless, their health had been the target of public health and local municipal policies. Despite this, women's health remained appallingly bad, with long-term morbidity and disability as consequences of pregnancies and childbirth (Spring Rice 1939).

Eugenicist ideas were frequently at the heart of many policies and women were still predominantly defined in terms of their identity as mothers, and children as future citizens. But there had been constructed in these years the semblance of a modern mass society. Social policies based upon future planning had been enacted in slum clearance schemes, health education, and localised welfare provision. It was still a deeply divided society economically and socially but it was more democratic and knowledgeable and, in a way, more controlled and organised. Porter sums up this change in his description of the target of policies:

> In the inter-war years Mr and Mrs Average and their children were becoming the focus of public medicine and health policies. (Porter 1999:644)

The desire to produce a more healthy and fit nation necessitated addressing the population as members of society, as citizens and not just individuals. Increasingly families and communities were seen as the basic structures of society, as molecules which together made up the total. One example of this trend of thinking was the Peckham Health Centre that was established in 1935 (Pearce and Crocker 1943). The Centre functioned as a club and a health centre. Families paid a small weekly subscription and were given periodic health checks and had access to all the leisure facilities including a swimming pool, classes and a weekly dance. Full nursery facilities were available for small children. Families were the target of research and surveillance but received social and community support. In many ways, this experiment was the embodiment of the fusing of social science, epidemiology and medicine which was to become a feature of the postwar period.

Although there had been measures to improve housing and education during this period, it was the continuation of poverty that mitigated against the universal improvement in health. Indeed, McGonigle and Kirby (1936) had shown that the health of families moving to new council estates actually worsened because of the extra rent which had to be paid at the expense of food. Clearly, what was needed was a complete overhaul of the social economic system; poverty, housing, education, employment all needed to be addressed in order to improve national health. The culture and structure of society in 1939 was radically different to that of hundred years previously. State intervention had grown and definitions of health and its importance to a society had also changed. Health had to a degree become the responsibility of government. But this entailed the surveillance and control of areas of social life previously outside of civil society and policies.

Public health legislation of the nineteenth and early twentieth centuries had been concerned to control infectious diseases, provide basic sanitation and curtail the worst aspects of rapid industrialisation. Incarceration and physical surveillance of the pauperised and the mentally and physically 'unfit' and 'degenerate' had been implemented, backed by beliefs in national efficiency and productivity. This was set against the increasing international competition between Britain and economic competitors.

Under the impact of Capitalist industrial development the relationship between the state and individuals changed. Instead of directing attention to social spaces and sites, the emphasis in public health turned to that of individual bodies. The bodies of children, women and men became a subject for surveillance, so too did their minds and behaviour.

The model of 'the family' came to be an organising principle and legislation on children's health and welfare became a part of the focus upon infant and, to a lesser extent, maternal welfare. The family became subjected to the public gaze of legislators, medical professionals, health visitors and welfare workers.

The concerns of the period have been categorised by Dean (1999:xvii) as those of maintaining 'physical efficiency', first by better sanitation of public spaces and then by the monitoring, surveillance and improvement of human bodies. We propose to adopt Dean's theory that this was just the first phase and was to be succeeded by the second, that of 'social efficiency' in the postwar welfare state.

CHAPTER 2

The Welfare State, Social Democracy and the Nation's Health

Introduction

During the period following the foundation of the post Second World War welfare state, the responsibility for procuring a healthy nation became a part of the role of the state. In this chapter we will be tracing the place of health within three distinctive overarching political discourses. It is important to note that these do not follow a strict chronological order. Elements of one political-cultural discourse can be seen to exist in a previous and a successive one. A specific concern can at one time be marginalised and at another be central, but can be seen to be permanently in existence.

The three distinct political discourses present during this period of time may be outlined as:

- Social democracy and welfarism
- Consumerism and individualism
- Communitarianism and social inclusion

Each of these political discourses was focused on a responsibility for health but varied in definition, approach and organisation. In some ways these can be seen as cultural zones within which policies on health and welfare provision are constructed.

The predominance of *social democracy and welfarism* was illustrated by the creation of the health service, the pre-eminence of hospital-based medicine and power of the medical profession and the decline of public health. Welfare services grew and the strong economy was based upon full male employment and the existence of a 'cradle to grave' welfare state. But it also meant that some groups were increasingly marginalised and excluded from full citizenship.

The discourse of *consumerism and individualism*, defined health as a consumer good to be attained by individual effort. Health became a personal responsibility and ill health was seen as largely preventable by avoidance of risk. Market values of efficiency and value for money were imposed upon the organisation of the health service but there was also a reaction against the hospital or institution as the preferred site of health and social care provision.

Under a *communitarian* discourse, the health and well-being of communities are currently seen as a result of joint responsibility between government and individuals. Whilst the responsibility of government is defined as providing the structures for health it is then the social responsibility of the individual to use the provision.

This chapter is concerned with the impact of these three different 'stages' of health and welfare provision during this period on the changing roles and purpose of community nursing. As well as these three stages within which changes took place, there were also discourses that entered into public discussion and directed much of the practices of community nurses. Before looking in depth at the differing stages of provision and at the discourses that accompanied them, it is important to firstly elaborate upon the ideas about the changing focus on the body and its efficiency with which we ended the previous chapter. Ellis (2000), has introduced this very important definition of the changing focus upon the human body which accompanied the successive development of health and welfare provision in Britain from the nineteenth century until the present. The period of Edwardian reforms, with the focus upon the 'physical efficiency' of bodies, as we have seen, was characterised by policies on physical and mental 'fitness' which further separated and then incarcerated those who did not measure up to specific standards. The discourse on efficiency was focused upon children, women as mothers and men as workers and soldiers. It was imbued with eugenicist ideas of selective breeding, underpinned by fears of a low birth rate and high infant mortality. The next stage involved the focus upon 'social efficiency' that began in the interwar years but accompanied the state provision of health and welfare in the postwar welfare state. This, in turn, was to be succeeded by the next stage, that of the 'independent body' (Ellis 2000:13). This stage was indicated by the policies of the mid 1970s onwards with the focus upon the individual body and the personal responsibility of individuals for their own health and well-being. We would also suggest that this stage can be seen to be in process of change to that of 'community efficiency' which is now becoming the focus of policies and strategies.

To summarise, we would argue that there are three dominant discourses of governmentality and health within which policies and directions of community nursing in the postwar period have been enacted. Within these overarching political-cultural discourses, specific discourses on 'health' or 'welfare' have also directed policies and practice. Social democracy focused upon the 'social efficiency' of bodies, consumerism upon the 'individual body' and communitarianism upon the 'community efficiency' of the body.

Social democracy and social efficiency

During the interwar years, the focus upon the physical efficiency of individuals within the population began to give way to a focusing upon the 'social efficiency' of the mass of society. The proposals for a national health service, the implementation of state measures to improve the health of children in deprived areas, the creation of 'new' industries, and the experiment of the Peckham Health Centre are all illustrations of this cultural shift. The social efficiency of the whole society was not defined solely in physical terms but also increasingly in psychological and emotional ones. As Armstrong has noted,

> In the mass society to develop in the inter-war years, the identification of the space between bodies as 'social' made possible a politics of the social. (Armstrong 1983:40)

This concern with social efficiency necessarily entailed more sophisticated mechanisms of surveillance. The family as a basic social group became the social body to be screened, surveilled and controlled. Notions of pathology became more widely applied so that people were screened for potential risk rather than for actual illnesses. This destroyed the 'old distinction between those who were healthy and those who were diseased' (Armstrong 1983:37). The new ideas of 'social medicine' placed the causation of diseases of both body and mind within a social space. Disease and illness could be seen to have socio-psychological causes. Therefore, it followed that people sharing a geographical space or a socio-economic space could be predicted to share a predisposition to certain diseases or illnesses and even dysfunctional social behaviour. Surveys and screening were the techniques used to ascertain the potentiality for 'risk'. This was already a trend before the advent of the Second World War but the foundation of the postwar welfare state and health service brought the whole population into the 'community gaze'.

The period of the focus upon 'social efficiency' during which the health of the nation became an accepted part of government organisation and responsibility can be divided into two distinct phases. The first phase might be described as one of optimism and confidence in the ability of government to deliver health and welfare as a social service, this was the 'high noon' of welfarism that immediately followed from the foundation of the NHS in 1948 and lasted until the early 1960s. The second phase, which began in the 1960s and lasted until the 1980s, we would define as still belonging to the social democratic-social efficiency discourse but one which increasingly showed signs of concern and doubt over the organisation and efficacy of the health service to deliver universal care in an equitable way. Within these two phases there also existed powerful discourses that shaped policies and had significance for the organisation and structure of the health services and role of community nursing.

The dominance of social democracy as a guiding principle coupled with the objective of social efficiency underpinned the foundation of the welfare state in Britain after 1945 (see Table 2.1). Although ideas of a planned economy which would offer order and stability as well as security for all citizens was in existence before the war, the victory in 1945 meant that Britain was to fully embrace the ideal of a welfare state. Within this, the provision of health care

Table 2.1   Landmarks of legislation: health and social welfare 1945–1979

1946	Family Allowance Act – allowance for every child under 16 except for first born, payable to mother
1946	National Insurance Act – national insurance scheme extended to include unemployment benefit, sickness, maternity, retirement pension, widows benefit National Health Service Act – free and universal access to medical care at point of need. Organised under 3 national services – GPs, local health authorities (including district nursing, health visiting and home helps), hospitals Mental Welfare departments for the education, training, supervision and care of mentally ill and handicapped people in residential homes and 'in' the community.
1948	National Assistance Act – complementary provsion for those not adequately covered by national insurance. Means-tested benefits to top up universal provision. Welfare departments set up, Part 111 of Act places duty on local authorities to provide residential accommodation for elderly and infirm, and temporary accommodation for 'urgent need'. Non-residential services also to be provided for disabled
1949	Housing Act – local authority housing provision on basis of need
1953	Guillebaud Committee reports on NHS costs – recommends more 'care in the community'
1954	Bradbeer Report highlights the conflict existing between occupational groups in NHS as detrimental to efficiency
1962	Hospital Plan recommends run down of long-stay hospitals, and building of large District General Hospitals for acute care, outpatient services
1962	Local Authorities develop own meals on wheels services
1964	Housing Corporation founded to fund and monitor housing associations
1965	Rent Act – principle of 'fair rents' in private lettings
1966	Ministry of Social Security Act – Supplementary benefit replaced national assistance. Means-tested system with more stringent rules. Higher rate paid to elderly claimants
1968	Seebohm Report – recommends amalgamation of Welfare, Mental Welfare and Children's departments into unified department
1970	Local Authority Social Services Act – creates social services departments. Home help services transferred to social services
1971	Social Security Act – introduction of Family Income Supplement (FIS) Means-tested to target low-paid working families.
1977	Housing (Homeless Persons Act) – defines statutory homelessness and gives priority to vulnerable groups, children. Responsibility of local authorities to house homeless in area
1979	Royal Commission on NHS – rejects the feasibility of shifting the responsibility for provision of care onto local authorities. Endorsement of existing system

was paramount. The type of health service which Britain adopted was based upon access to medical expertise rather than a collectivist public health approach (Klein 1989). The NHS was based upon the premise that there should be social equality in gaining access to medical, nursing and hospital services;

> every man, woman and child can rely on getting all the advice and treatment and care which they need...and that what they get shall be the best medical and other facilities available. (1944 White Paper cited in Klein 1989:10)

The creation of the NHS under the guidance of Aneurin Bevan split an already divided medical profession into two distinct interest groups. The 'battle with the doctors' (Webster 1991, Timmins 1996), resulted in the formal organisation of the service being somewhat of a 'compromise solution' (Allsop 1984), with a split between the hospital service and general practice. But undoubtedly the health service prioritised the hospital consultant and established hospital-based health care as of paramount importance. The nationalisation of hospitals that had taken place at the outset of war in 1940 under the Emergency Medical Service, meant that the overall organisation and funding of this hospital service became a part of the new centralised welfare state.

The Beveridge Plan (Beveridge 1942) which was the blueprint of the welfare state contained not only the determination to tackle the 'five giants' of poverty, disease, want, ignorance and idleness, it also reflected the beliefs and attitudes of the time. The creation of a welfare state to make accessible to everyone a lifetime of security and freedom from extreme poverty and want, involved state action across many fronts. This universal accessibility was the essence of social democracy, not the actual management and control of the provision of health and social welfare. For many, the connection between social democracy and universal citizenship was made through the construction of the welfare state. But the welfare state was also founded upon a set of ideas and beliefs. Among these was a specific model of the 'normal' family and the gendered roles of men and women.

The direction of policies on health and on welfare diverged quite dramatically. The National Health Service was essentially placed in the public sphere of hospitals and institutions. Nurses and medical students were trained in hospitals even if they were to pursue a career in the community. Health care was centralised and bureaucratised into large state institutions and organisations. District nursing, mental nursing and even school nursing was unambiguously placed within the public sphere of the NHS.

Welfare and social care on the other hand, became increasingly based within the private sphere of the family. The focus upon the child became more pronounced as the social effects of the war became visible (see Table 2.2). The new professionalised social workers based their practice upon the individual family within the casework approach where the influence of new psychological theories were central. Health visiting was caught in a pincer movement between the basis of training within the health service and practice in the private sphere of the family.

Social efficiency and the discourse of the 'problem' family

The Beveridge Plan had, at its heart, a specific model of 'the family' based upon the economic contribution of men and the financial dependency of women. It must also be remembered that the existing fears of a low birth rate that had been a feature of the interwar years were still strong and a pro-natalist stance was very much a part of the new provisions for social insurance

Table 2.2   State and the welfare of children and the family 1940–2000

1940	Pacifist Service Units formed to help evacuees and bombed out families
1943	Women's Group of Public Welfare publishes report 'Our Towns' which uses phrase 'problem families'
1945	Family Allowance Act – benefit paid to mother for second and subsequent children only
1946	The Care of Children Committee (Curtis Report) on death of Denis O'Neill aged 12, when in foster care. Foster parents jailed
1948	Children Act – Children's Departments created as part of Social Services. Growth of social work speciality of care and protection of children. Covers children in care, as well as in family
1948	Nurseries and Child-Minders Regulation Act – statutory duty of local authorities to supervise nurseries and minders
1949	Adoption of Children Act – followed 1939 legislation, registration of adoption societies, restriction on sending children abroad, consent must be unconditional, continuous supervision of child until school-leaving age
1963	Children and Young Persons Act – family service for disturbed families. Link between delinquency and deprivation in families
1972	Child benefit paid to mother for all children under age of 16
1975	Children Act – facilitated the right of removal of children from 'natural' family if suspected of abuse or neglect. Followed from death of Maria Colwell when returned to family
1976	Court Report on child health services. Link between ill health and mortality with socio-economic class made clear
1985	Publication of official report into death of Jasmine Beckford – highly critical of social work practice
1986	Family Credit benefit introduced – claimed by working parents who earned lower than average income. Paid to mainly mothers. Benefits withdrawn from 16–18 year olds living in family home
1987	Cleveland crisis – the medical diagnosis of existence of child abuse on large scale involved removal of many children from own homes
1988	Butler-Sloss report on Cleveland – argues for more cooperation between social workers, police, health services and support for parents
1989	Children Act – role of parents strengthened. Rights and welfare of the child to be of primary importance
1990	Child Support Act – 'absent' fathers pursued for maintenance of child even after divorce/separation. Mother to name father of child
1998	Welfare to Work programme – single mothers 'encouraged' to take up work. Child care allowances made
1998	Supporting Families – Consultative document – recommends family-friendly employment policies, welfare to work, implementation of early intervention projects
1999	Criminal Justice Act – curfews enforceable on children under 10. Truancy from school – families to be fined after persistent offending
1999	Working Families Tax Credit replaces Family Credit tax exemptions and allowances paid by employer, not as a state benefit. Guaranteed weekly income to families in work

and welfare. A famous passage from the Beveridge Report clearly sets out the role of the family and especially of women, in the future society;

> During marriage most women will not be gainfully employed . . . . In the next thirty years housewives as mothers have vital work to do in ensuring the adequate continuance of the British race. (Beveridge 1942:53)

This phrase clearly set the structure for the postwar society, based upon gendered divisions. Within this model, family women traded housework, childbirth and child rearing and physical and emotional caring in return for economic support (Finch and Groves 1983). The role of men was to be workers and to keep their dependents from the necessity of claiming from the state. This focus upon the role of motherhood was an extension of that which prevailed at the beginning of the century. Motherhood now was not only charged with the responsibility for the physical survival of children but also for their emotional and psychological development and socialisation into citizenship. But what of those families who did not 'fit' the model?

The discourse of the 'problem family' emerged early on during the war when evacuation of children and mothers from the overcrowded urban industrial areas to rural areas took place. Although the fear of pauperism of the 'residium' had been in existence a century before, the new discourse was based upon the new visibility of this group. A stunning passage in the report on evacuation sums up this feeling;

> The effect of evacuation was to flood the dark places with light and bring home to the national consciousness that the 'submerged tenth' described by Charles Booth still exists in our towns like a hidden sore, poor, dirty and crude in its habits, an intolerable and degrading burden to decent people forced by poverty to neighbour with it. Within this group are the 'problem families', always on the edge of pauperism and crime, riddled with mental and physical defects, in and out of the Courts for child neglect, a menace to the community. (Womens Group on Public Welfare 1943: Introduction)

During the early stages of the war when bombing of towns and cities was at its height, it was a religious voluntary group which first took up the challenge of the 'rehabilitation' of such families. The Pacifist Service Units (PSUs) founded in Liverpool and Manchester in 1940, worked with bombed out families in areas of high risk and deprivation. A report of their work (Stephens 1945) laid stress on the multi-causal nature of such dereliction and the need for practical material help as well as understanding and support. But, even here, a Foreword by Rowntree talks of the problem of the 'subnormal' family that 'will have to be faced with improved standards of welfare'. (Stephens 1945:1)

By 1947, the work of the PSU had been amalgamated into the welfare state and became the province of Family Service Units within the sphere of social services. Volunteers became paid workers and by 1950 were trained with health visitor students. New categories of 'problem families' became defined (McKie 1963:28), such as 'baffling families' who were of 'low mentality', with bad health, poverty, father unemployed, 'children over-protected and timid, parents uncooperative and demanding' with bad school attendance. The work of health visitors with the 'problem families' expanded as did the categories of need. A text book on health visiting illustrated the types to be dealt with; the 'broken family', 'the incomplete family', as well as the 'abnormal family' (McEwan 1951:93–4). Broken and incomplete families were to be treated with understanding and suggestions for counselling and support, especially to unmarried mothers. The role of the health visitor was now verging upon that of social worker, and by 1960 the largest number of referrals to the Family Service Units was made by health visitors (McKie 1963:82).

The focus by the state upon the welfare of children now stretched beyond the narrow range of the school health services into support and treatment for those 'disadvantaged' from birth, to encompass the necessity of 'social adjustment' into society. Policies on the protection of children, often inspired and illustrated by an individual tragedy, such as the death of 10 year old Dennis O'Neil in foster care in 1945, highlighted the new responsibility of the state. But this responsibility was matched by the citizen's responsibility to engage in a reciprocal relationship. Children had to be socialised into social conformity and law-abiding behaviour. Juvenile delinquency became a prominent and publicised concern in postwar society. The influence of psychology was noticeable in the defined causes of the 'maladjusted' child (Stott 1956). Within this paradigm the influence of the 'maternal deprivation' theories of Bowlby (1953) had great influence on the training of social workers and health visitors. Within the education system the application of IQ tests gave a scientific gloss to existing beliefs in the 'low mentality' of the 'slum-breakdown family' which by the mid 1950s included certain 'immigrant' families with 'medieval domestic hygiene' (Stott 1956:57).

The focus upon the protection, socialisation and monitoring of the child in social policies replaced to a certain extent the focus upon physical health and well-being. The child became a potential victim of uncaring parents, inadequate socialisation and the state. The physical health of children and adults was the responsibility of the NHS that, by 1948, organised all branches of community nursing.

Organisation and practice of community nursing in welfarism

The organisation of the NHS in 1948 had profound consequences for the placing of community nursing within the sphere of public health. The domination of medical services in the health service meant that the role of public health diminished. Consequently, 'public health became a rag bag of activities' (Lewis 1986:11). After 1948, public health departments relinquished administration of the municipal hospitals and remained responsible only for environmental issues, notification of infectious diseases and maternal and child health.

The tripartite organisation consisted of varying hierarchies of power, the hospitals were dominated by consultants, the local practices by GPs and the local authorities with local Medical Officers of Health in a greatly reduced role. What of community nursing in this structure?

The organisation of district nursing was radically altered with the NHS in 1948. As a history of the period illustrates (Stocks 1960:171), the advent of an 'admittedly socialist government' was to break the existing tie between home nursing and voluntary associations. Local authorities were now required to provide 'nurses to attend persons requiring nursing in their own homes, free of charge' (Stocks 1960:172), thus eradicating the old methods of judging the 'deserving' nature of the sick. There were protacted negotiations over the following years between the voluntary associations, the Queens Institute and the local authorities over the training, payment and supply of district nursing services. But the sweep of welfare reform meant that district nurses became paid employees of the state whose main function was that of nursing the sick. In some ways, their role became narrowed as the emphasis was placed upon the delivery of medical and health services with aspects of social welfare being diverted to other occupations. District nursing, unlike health visiting, was a hidden occupation, it was marginal to the direction of technologically determined and hospital-based health policy during and immediately after the war (Dingwall et al. 1988:197). Its practice was also narrowed to the provision of nursing services, primarily to the elderly sick in their own homes, but the provision of social care and 'education' of families was now placed elsewhere.

The discourse of the 'problem family' enveloped the expansion and high profile of health visiting in the postwar welfare state, but this also added to the contradictions inherent within the practice itself. Health visiting was positioned between health and social care and did not 'belong' totally in either sphere. The connection between health visiting and social work became more pronounced with the emphasis upon child welfare. Although officially the work of the health visitor as set out in the 1946 White Paper (McEwan 1951:25) covered a range of activities including that of TB visitor and inspector of institutions for mentally deficient children, nevertheless the focus was upon working with pre-school children and mothers in the private sphere of the home. The postwar concerns about juvenile delinquency and unmarried mothers also informed health visiting practice. The Jameson Report (MoH 1956), clearly set out the new responsibilities of health visitors; the focus was on 'health education and social advice' with collaboration with other professionals including social workers, GPs, and hospital almoners. Health visitors were to pay special regard to 'mental hygiene of children and play a part in the child guidance service. This extension of practice meant that it was calculated that more health visitors would have to be recruited given a set ratio of visits needed per area, and there was also a recommendation that the recruitment base should be widened to included non-nurses (MoH 1956:xii–xiii).

The momentum over child welfare also pushed school nursing into the centre of policies. The Education Act of 1944 made the setting up of a school health service a statutory requirement imposed upon all education authorities. The school nurse (often called the school health visitor) had to hold health visiting qualifications and was responsible for assisting at routine medical inspections, assessment of nutrition, grading of children on 'fitness' and hygiene, carrying out vision and hearing tests and foot clinics. She was also responsible for vermin control and so was often referred to as the 'nit lady', and for health education including sex education for girls. This latter role had also been stressed by the report on evacuation (Womens Group on Public Welfare 1943), where the school nurse was described as the ideal person to give advice on menstruation and sexual behaviour.

The war had also promoted the employment of medical and health services in industry. In 1940, the Factories (Medical and Welfare Services) Order meant that doctors and nurses were employed in large factories to oversee not just health and welfare but also to provide ambulance services. Courses for industrial nursing were started and funded by the Royal College of Nursing (RCN). Industrial nursing became a very popular field of public service (Charley 1978). Following from the foundation of the NHS, an industrial nursing service was introduced in the newly nationalised industries of coal, railways, on the docks as well as in areas of high female employment. Nurses ran first aid courses as well as monitoring infectious diseases and industrial accidents. The ideas of social democracy that underpinned much of the nationalisation programme coupled with full employment which followed in postwar era, meant that this was the highpoint of the industrial nursing service.

Mental nursing, however, remained in the shadows. The mental health services 'were initially largely unaffected by the introduction of the NHS' (Dingwall et al. 1988:135). The interest of local authorities and the popular appeal of the hospital services meant that mental institutions were starved of investment and continued to 'moulder away in antiquated buildings' (Webster 1988:325). As elsewhere in the health service, medical domination was paramount in the diagnosis and treatment of mental illness and disorders. The medical model of mental illness meant that treatment was placed within an institution and subject to little regulation. But the restraint of patients by use of medication and tranquilising drugs grew from the early 1950s onwards. This meant that stays in institutions tended towards the short term. From the mid 1950s onwards, there was a dramatic decrease in admissions to mental hospitals, reversing the trend since the foundation of the asylum system in the nineteenth century. In 1951, the Royal College of Psychiatrists was founded (replacing the Royal Medico-Psychological Association), and the examinations for mental nursing were taken over by the GNC.

Mental nursing thus became a branch of generalist nursing at the same time as psychiatry gained in status and reward. Some mental disorders now appeared to be in the realm of the 'treatable' or even 'curable'. However, mental nursing did not share in this new-found status, and disputes over pay and conditions were common throughout the late 1940s and 1950s. In 1946 COHSE (Confederation of Health Service Employees) replaced the NASW (National Association of Social Workers) as the trade union representing mental nurses. 'The medicalization of the asylums and their reconceptualization as hospitals, reconstituted custodial attendants as nurses for the mentally sick and the defective' (Dingwall et al. 1988:143).

The National Health Service within the overall adoption of welfarism and the welfare state was based upon the delivery of medical services that would effect cures. This meant, of necessity, that those groups suffering from the 'incurable' disorders of mental disorder and old age were assigned a relatively low status. The so-called Cinderella services were still not given parity in the social democratic welfare state. The emphasis on the productive citizen and on child welfare had led to the further exclusion of specific groups from the general improvement that the welfare reforms had brought. This exclusion led to a powerful discourse of the following period of social democracy and welfarism during the 1960s.

The backlash against institutionalisation

Concern over the plight of those who were not included in the general improvement in health services surfaced almost from the start of the NHS. Various pressure groups such as Help the Aged, MIND and Mencap were founded in 1946, to press for recognition and better services for the 'Cinderella' groups. But the demographic changes and the services required by these groups were vastly different.

The poverty of working-class elderly people was obvious from the beginning of the welfare state when the largest percentage of those claiming National Assistance were revealed to be pensioners. Those who became eligible for pensions in 1946, had of course been born in the nineteenth century and many had suffered from a legacy of poverty, ill health and neglect. But for others, the NHS and the welfare provisions in general began to contribute to an increase in life expectancy. By the early 1960s, there was already talk of an 'ageing population' and the future demands of the elderly upon the health services were being defined as a problem. The needs of elderly people required many agencies as well as health, notably housing and social services (Jones 1994). Community services were inadequate and the role of caring for an elderly relative fell to wives, daughters and daughters-in-law to perform unpaid and in the hidden setting of the home. There was an expansion of home help services, meals-on-wheels and day clubs, but the picture was patchy. Some local authorities began building sheltered housing in the early 1960s but there was not a mass national programme. The other alternative for the care of frail elderly people without family or formal support, was, as it had always been, institutionalisation. The inadequate provision of community services for this expanding number meant that residential accommodation had to be increased (Webster 1988). The adaptation of 'grossly unsuitable accommodation inherited from the Poor Law authorities' (Webster 1988:376) took place after 1948, with the building of purpose-built units very much in the minority. The conditions in many of these 'homes' became the subject of press speculation but they were seen as a preferable alternative to the occupation of hospital beds. In 1967, the publication of a damning report (Townsend 1962), contained an appalling catalogue of abuse, neglect and cruelty in many of the residential units. This was based upon the testimony of nurses and social workers working with elderly people in institutions. The following year, local authorities had the statutory duty to provide home help services to all elderly people in their area who were judged in need. But if treatment of elderly people gained a higher profile, it was eclipsed by the scandals which overtook mental hospitals.

The backlash against the institutions had in fact officially begun in 1961 when Enoch Powell, the Health Minister, had stunned a meeting of the National Association for Mental Health when he described the existing mental institutions as 'rising unmistakably and daunting out of the countryside – the asylums which our forefathers had built with such immense solidity' (quoted in Timmins 1996:211).

In the field of child welfare, the person of the individual child has often been symbolically used to effect change, as in the case of Dennis O'Neil and Jasmine Beckford among others. In the field of mental health it was the conditions in the long stay mental institutions which attached attention and criticism. The scandal at Ely hospital which involved accusations of brutality and neglect towards patients was focused upon and reported in sensational detail in the popular press in the late 1960s, and culminated in a damning public inquiry in 1969. This was one case among others taking place in Farleigh, Whittington, South Ockenden, but it was Ely that captured the headlines and became a symbol of the continuing existence of the Victorian asylum. Timmins (1996:258), also argues that the current postwar images of concentration camps were also utilised in the picture of neglect and horror.

The growing criticism of the inadequacies and loopholes of the welfare state spread to other spheres in the relatively affluent period of the 1960s and 1970s. The 're-discovery of poverty' (Abel-Smith and Townsend 1965), the plight of the homeless illustrated by the television drama 'Cathy Come Home' in 1966, and the setting up of campaigning groups like Shelter and Child Poverty Action Group, all added to the atmosphere of unease and concern. After only twenty years, the welfare state was being subjected to scrutiny and criticism, mostly by the political left who felt that it had not fulfilled its promise of a 'cradle to grave' society for all. But there was still a belief in social democracy and in the primary role for the state in the delivery of services. Social work too had undergone a transformation after the Seebohm Report of 1968 and social work departments were expanded. But the seeds of doubt were there, and moves to re-organise the NHS and make it more efficient and democratic took place.

Reorganisation and the impact on community nursing

The costs of the NHS, far from diminishing as predicted by Beveridge, were spiralling, and the Guillebaud Committee had been charged with the investigation of costs in 1953. Although the Committee found that overall the service gave good value for money, the Report, published in 1956 (MoH 1956), recommended that more care should be placed out of the hospital system and into the community. Despite this, the NHS continued to be primarily, in Klein's words 'a hospital service' (Klein 1989:7). The emphasis on hospital services remained paramount even though ideas of more community-based care were beginning to be aired. In 1962, the Hospital Plan was revealed by the Minister of Health, Enoch Powell. The majority of Britain's hospitals had been built in the last century and the Plan was for a massive hospital building programme centred on the large District General Hospital and the closing of small community or cottage hospitals. Despite his intention to close down the mental asylums, the enthusiasm for the building of high-tech large hospitals was unabated. At the same time as community-based care was being recommended for the elderly and for people with mental disorders, hospital admission for the 'curable' was increasing. The shortage of beds and shortage of nursing staff was a major problem. Nurse recruitment was stepped up with Powell initiating the setting up of employment agencies recruiting nurses from the Caribbean and other previous outposts of the British empire.

Nursing was affected by a series of measures throughout the 1960s and 1970s; in 1966 the Salmon Report sought to modernise the organisation of nursing and abolished the post of matron, the Mayston Report in 1969 brought management structures to community nursing and the Briggs Report in 1972 recommended a system of further education for nurses. These were all attempts to streamline and modernise nursing in order to fit in with the projected plans for a large and high-tech hospital service. The emphasis was on hospital nursing, however, with community nursing playing a subordinate role. It must be stressed that ever since regulation in 1919, community nursing has always been seen as a post-hospital experience, all community nurses have been trained and socialised into the hospital system prior to work in the community. There were, however, changes to the organisation and structure of branches within community nursing with the reorganisation of the health service and local government in 1974.

The reorganisation of the health service in 1974 had far-reaching effects on health visiting especially. The restructuring included the increase in democratic accountability by the setting up of Community Health Councils, the inclusion of trade union representatives on health authorities but, importantly, it also involved the shift for the responsibility of health visitor services from local authority control to the health service. Health centres were established and multi-partnered GP practices began to replace the traditional single-handed GP.

The 1974 restructuring also further decreased the status and importance of public health. The post of Medical Officer of Health disappeared and was replaced by that of community physician who retained the responsibility for maternal and infant welfare only. Environmental health shifted from public health into the local authority control of Environment Health Officers who were not health professionals.

The ambiguity of health visiting practice and its relationship to social work was now visible and attempts were made by the profession to clearly define health visiting duties. The Seebohm Report on social work in 1968 had been dismissive of the contribution of health visiting to social problems. The two occupations had set up two distinct qualifying bodies in 1962, but the ambiguities remained (Dingwall 1975). The move to place health visiting firmly within primary health care was literally taken after 1974 when health visitors were formally 'attached' to GP practices. This was not always an easy transition, as Dingwall (1974) reported, with many GPs being totally ignorant of the role and responsibilities of health visitors and inclined to regard them as nurses or almoners.

The Council for Education and Training of Health Visitors (CETHV) set out the defining principles of practice in 1977, where the search for health needs was emphasised as well as the educative function and work with 'the family'. But health visiting was in rather an identity vacuum with the expansion of social work on the one hand and the emphasis in community-based care moving towards the elderly and the mentally ill.

District nurses, on the other hand, appeared to be in a favourable organisational and demographic position. District nurses were employed solely by health authorities after 1974, and the need for training had been emphasised in the Briggs Report. The increase in the elderly population appeared to signal an increased demand for services, but this was nursing which required low technological input and as such did not receive high recognition (Dingwall et al. 1988:203).

Mental nursing had come from the shadows by the mid 1970s but this transition was problematic. The asylum system was in disrepute and the much quoted adage that 'the worst home is better than the best mental hospital' (Cummings 1957:55) appeared to be the future guiding principle of policy. The publication in 1975 of the Better Services for the Mentally Ill report, stressed the future transition to community care but also gave an assurance that the old hospitals would not be precipitously run down. But the contraction of the mental hospitals had begun and the training of mental nurses now emphasised the community and therapeutic nature of practice. But the move was slow, and in 1977 there was still only about 1000 community psychiatric nurses (CPNs) compared with 50,000 working in hospitals (DHSS 1980: 49–50). In contrast, services for those with a mental handicap (especially children) fared better. The number of community nurses in mental handicap increased during the same time from 50 to 300 (DHSS 1979–81:23).

This differential could be explained by the fact that the services to mentally handicapped children were the focus of change within the overall momentum on child welfare.

In many ways, the retreat from a custodial service to one of therapy and community care meant that mental nursing, like health visiting, became an ambiguous practice. The Jay Report in 1979 on mental handicap care, recommended the setting up of small local units staffed by a new group of care workers qualified in social work. In effect 'nursing was invited to abandon the territory awarded to it in 1919 in favour of social work' (Dingwall et al. 1988:141).

By the 1970s, it was clear that much of the apolitical consensus regarding the welfare state and the NHS had begun to crack. The health service had moved from being 'above politics' to being a part of all political agendas. Society had also undergone great changes (which we will examine in detail in Chapter 3) and these placed further strain upon the ideal of a mass society provided for by the universalist welfare state. The focus on 'social efficiency' was being confronted by a new political-cultural discourse that placed more importance upon the 'individual body' and on the redefining of the citizen as a consumer.

Individualism, the market and consumerism

The criticism of the welfare state's ability to deliver a coherent system of health and social care within a democratic society which had been first articulated by the political left in the 1960s and 70s, was echoed by those of the New Right. But the solution proffered was of a radically different nature. The political-cultural philosophy that emerged and gained in hegemony throughout the 1980s was a hybrid of past and present economic and moral beliefs. An early publication (Joseph and Sumption 1979) made clear that its main tenets were the primacy of the individual over the collective, freedom of choice within a market system and the 'rolling back of the state'. This phrase was to become a central organising principle of all the reforms of public services throughout the following decade. The election of Margaret Thatcher as prime minister at the head of a radical Conservative administration in 1979, gave the term Thatcherism to the direction and range of policies dedicated to the breaking away from the 'nanny state'.

Within this moral crusade, the public services and state-owned industries were seen as inefficient, undemocratic and costly. The remedy was to apply the discipline of the market and the values and organisation of private industry. Nationalised industries and public utilities such as gas, electricity and telecommunications were privatised and shares sold off to investors in a massive programme to promote 'popular capitalism'. But the privatisation of other forms of public services such as education, social security and especially the health service proved rather more problematic. 'For the Thatcherites, the constraints, both circumstantial and self-imposed, which they faced meant that a shift to a full-blown market economy was both politically and socially untenable' (Moon 1997:113).

The National Health Service held a special place in the lexicon of British social democracy. Funded by taxation and contributory insurance payments, the health service was used and depended upon by a large section of the middle class and a complete privatisation of the service would have been particularly politically unsustainable. However, the dominant values of efficiency and cost effectiveness were to be brought to the organisation of the

NHS that still retained its fundamental principle of being free at the point of need. If the health service could not be taken to market then the market would be taken to the health service.

The project to make the health service more competitive and efficient through the application of an internal market system was at the centre of policies throughout the 1980s. The creation of the quasi-market (Bartlett 1991, Bartlett and Le Grand 1993), meant that the internal market could operate within the strict boundaries set by the central state. Under this set up, certain hotel services such as catering and cleaning were put to external competitive tendering and the separation of the purchasing and provision of services meant that individual GPs and hospitals could act as independent buyers and sellers. The essential nature of the health service as provider remained but the organisation of provision was placed within a 'managed market' (Enthoven 1985). This brought to prominence another phenomenon, the advent of professional managerialism which challenged the existing power hierarchy which had dominated the NHS since its foundation in 1948.

The relationship between the professionals and patients was clearly defined within the NHS at its inception, it has been characterised as 'a monument to enlightened paternalism' (Klein 1989:17). The medical profession dominated all areas of the NHS and the role of the patient was to be passive and grateful. It was this relationship that the New Right theorists felt to be a negation of the freedom of the individual. The identity of patient was to be replaced by that of an active consumer (North 1997). But this transition was a problematic one, for the real market did not exist so therefore a real consumerism was not possible. Instead of individuals operating as consumer/purchasers in their own interests within the quasi-market, designated groups of professionals purchased services on behalf of the individual. The new competitive system which pitched hospital against hospital in a bid to attract purchasers of services was unveiled in the government document *Working For Patients* (DoH 1989). In a Foreword, Margaret Thatcher summed up the philosophical objective of the system, 'to extend patient choice, delegate responsibility to where services are provided and secure the best value for money' (DoH 1989).

But it was not patients who were to be given the choice, GPs were offered the opportunity to become independent budget holders able to purchase services for 'their' patients from hospitals who were also locked in a competitive system where they vied with one another to offer cost-effective services. This quasi-consumerism meant that the NHS took on the dynamic but irrational and potentially anarchic elements of a market system. GPs were placed in competition with each other between fund-holders and non fund-holders, hospitals who became independent trusts were pitted against those who remained directly funded and the monolithic health service fragmented into competing units. But the health service itself remained under state control and funding. In order to preserve and improve efficiency, the imposition of a managerialist ethos was essential.

The necessity for better management of the NHS had been recognised in 1974, with the reorganisation and the widening of membership of District Health Authorities and hospital management boards. But the implementation of professional general management to the running of the NHS followed from the Griffiths report in 1983 (DHSS 1983). The appointment of Roy Griffiths, a director of the retail food chain of Sainsbury's, to chair an inquiry into management of the NHS, was in itself a revealing move. The importation of external business methods and values into a public service was a central part of government strategy. The health service was to be recreated as 'NHS plc' (Strong and Robinson 1990:3).

But the application of general management at every level of the service down to individual hospital units entailed the transformation of existing power structures based upon medical dominance. Nursing had adopted certain management structures since the 1970s but still, on the whole, remained subordinate to the powerful medical profession on a daily basis. 'Doctors would not be led. Nurses did not know how to lead' (Strong and Robinson 1990:65).

The challenge to the power of the professions posed by general management may be more of an ideological than an organisational one. Research has shown that, after the introduction of general management in 1984, both the medical and nursing professions attempted a strategy of inclusion (Harrison and Pollitt 1994). Many consultants became involved in clinical directorates and managed to retain a power to control medical audits (Gillespie 1997:101). Nursing, after initial opposition to the Report, 'rose from the ashes' (Klein 1989) and nurses were placed in charge of quality assurance programmes (Petchey 1986). Nevertheless, something fundamental had changed in the NHS, the acceptance by the clinical trades of targets, cost-effectiveness and efficiency meant that the service adopted a degree of market values and managerial direction.

This change also spread to the delivery of health services outside of the hospital service into general practice and community nursing. The new contract drawn up between the government and GPs was announced in 1990. This was to be imposed, without consultation, upon all GPs regardless of fund-holding status. The contract set targets for the immunisation of children, cervical screening programmes, the setting up of 'health promotion' clinics such as Well Woman Clinics and the carrying out of compulsory health checks on elderly patients. Payment was dependent upon the achievement of set percentages of completion of these targeted activities. The taking over of child health surveillance by GPs from the community-based health visitor service, was to create a degree of antagonism. The aim of the new contract was to make GPs accountable for the achievement of sections of service provision, it was 'health' defined as the provision of designated services. But it was just a part of a whole reworking of definitions of health and individual responsibility.

The promotion of health – an individualist discourse

Within the marketisation of the NHS, a redefining of health and the role of the individual body gained a philosophical hegemony. The body became an object of consumption and signifier of health; 'health is something which can be bought (by investment in private health care), sold (via health food stores and health centres) given (by surgery and drugs) and lost (following accident or disease)' (Aggleton 1990, quoted in Wilkinson 1995:982).

Health was also increasingly defined as being an individual responsibility. 'Take Care of Yourself' became the guiding principle which shifted from the realms of economic and social philosophy to health care. In the New Right political climate of the 1980s, the rising costs of health care provision promoted a concern to get people to take more responsibility for their own health either by purchasing private health care or by adopting a 'healthier' lifestyle.

Social inequalities in health, that had ironically been publicised in the first year of the first Thatcher administration by the Black Report (DHSS 1980a), were sidelined in the focus upon the role assigned to individual behaviour. As at the beginning of the century, the blame for infant mortality was put on the ignorance of mothers rather than on poverty, low wages and bad housing; so the blame for many degenerative diseases such as heart disease and cancers, was placed upon the ignorance of individuals. The concept of 'risky behaviour' was applied to smoking, drinking, lack of exercise and consumption of fatty and unhealthy food, and massive campaigns were launched to educate people into healthier lifestyles. The connection between ill health and poverty and the fact that the poorest were the most likely to have 'unhealthy' lifestyles was effectively overlooked in the dash to promote healthy living.

The political desire to move health care from an emphasis on cure to one of prevention began in 1976 with the policy discussion document *Prevention and Health: Everybody's Business* (DHSS 1976). This document also, however, highlighted social class and regional variations in health status, even if the basic message was one of the necessity for people to be 'educated' into making healthy choices. But it was in 1978, with the publication of the World Health Organisation's, 'Health For All' programme (WHO 1978), that the policies of health promotion really gained momentum. In 1986, the *Ottawa Charter for Health Promotion* (WHO 1986), defined health promotion as 'the process of enabling people to increase control over and improve their health'. It is this assumption, that 'people' regardless of their socio-economic status can 'gain control', which underlies critiques of such health promotion messages.

Critiques of the individualistic nature of health promotion pointed to its 'victim blaming' approach (Ashton and Seymour 1988) and posed instead a structural perspective that sought to improve a wide range of environmental and social conditions. Other writers argued that those whose social conditions rendered them vulnerable to diseases were also excluded from the benefits of an improved lifestyle (Blaxter 1990). Critics like McQueen (1988) argued that the individualistic emphasis of health promotion coincided exactly with the right-wing political orientation of most western governments during this period. Feminist writers (Daykin and Naidoo 1995) argued that the burden to promote not only their own health but that of 'all the family' fell mainly on women. But within a plethora of sociological criticism another issue was raised, that of the denial of the multi-factoral nature of disease.

The campaign to prevent heart disease was criticised by Davison et al. (1991) as a distortion of the truth which people recognised as such thereby causing them to reject the 'health messages' given by professionals:

> health education has never come to terms with the complex relationship between the individual and the collective in the field of health and illness. Rather it has opted for a form of worthy dishonesty based on . . . half truth, simplification and distortion. (Davison et al. 1991:16–17)

Health educators intent on promoting a healthy diet, were accused of being 'blind to the serious consequences of their propaganda' (Le Fanu 1986:124). Despite these criticisms it was clear that with the emphasis on prevention a new paradigm of health care had been formed. This involved an extension of the 'surveillance' techniques that Armstrong (1983) argues have been developed to monitor and control populations. The extension of monitoring, screening and the setting of targets and indicators of health have played a part in this greater employment of control mechanisms.

The new GP contract in 1990, which gave remuneration for the introduction of health promotion clinics, was mainly aimed at women and based upon cervical and breast screening, and children in the child surveillance and development clinics. Interestingly, although men are more at risk from heart disease and accidents as well as specific cancers, they have not been subjected to the same monitoring and surveillance techniques as women and children. Although it was GP practices that gained financially from the setting up of these services, it was actually practice nurses (employed by them) or health visitors who carried out the 'hands-on' work.

In 1992, the government set out distinct targets of 'health gain' to be achieved by the end of the century in the publication *The Health of the Nation* (DoH 1992). It was the achievement of these targeted reductions in smoking, obesity, heart diseases. cancers, mental illness and even accidents by which health authorities, Trusts, the medical profession and community nursing would be evaluated.

Within this move to a new paradigm of health can be seen a focus upon the individual rather than the social body. As Britain became a more socially and economically divided society throughout the 1980s and 1990s, the emphasis in health service provision centred upon the top-down definition of health gain. Despite evidence that illness was causally linked to poverty (Townsend et al. 1988, Wilkinson and Davey Smith 1989, Rowntree Foundation 1997), the thrust of policies and practice was upon the atomised individual. This was to have special impact upon the practice of health visiting.

'Whither health visiting?'

On the surface, the trends in health policy and service provision with the emphasis on health promotion, seemed to offer an enlarged role for health visiting. But the shift from a curative model of health to one of prevention, which should perhaps have signalled a new high profile position for health visiting, in fact formed the background to a period of crisis that extended until the late 1990s. Why did this happen?

We would suggest three main reasons; primarily it was because the restructuring of the health service was centred upon a GP-led and market-driven service; this in turn was to lead to the decline of a wider public health remit of local authorities; and finally, the change in direction of health policies caused changes in nurse education and forced health visiting to confront the question of its continued existence as an identifiable and autonomous service.

The change in focus from an 'illness service to a health service offering help to prevent disease and disability' which was the objective of the *Promoting Better Health* White Paper (DHSS 1987) was accompanied by the shift to a community-based but medically-led service. As the then leader of the RCN perceptively observed, the proposals of the White Paper were

> fundamentally concerned with medical services, not with primary health care.... General practice is still centre stage; district nurses and health visitors are confined to walk-on parts. (Clay 1988)

Interestingly, in 1986, the government commissioned Cumberlege Report (DHSS 1986) had proffered an alternative model of the organisation of community-based services in the setting up of neighbourhood nursing teams. These would be separate and autonomous groupings able to develop working agreements and contracts with GP practices. But, as Fatchett (1990), noted, this model was never to be a part of government policy, the health agenda of which was to lead to a 'dimunition in the role of community nursing and, in particular, in the role of the health visitor' (Fatchett 1990:216).

The centering of all aspects of primary health care delivery, including health promotion clinics and child health surveillance in the site of the GP surgery, further removed from health visitors an essential component of their occupational identity. This caused a great deal of publicised concern within health visiting especially the perceived danger that GPs would prefer to employ practice nurses to undertake this work thus further marginalising health visiting (Potrykus 1989). The relationship between health visiting and general practice became more tense and problematic following the advent of fundholding. The identification of the fundholder GP as a purchaser of services via contracts entered into with Community Health Trusts, health authorities and other organisations was set out in the NHS and Community Care Act (DHSS 1990). Within the ranks of health visiting, this prompted even more fears for its future existence and the Health Visitors' Association (HVA) supported a mass lobby of Parliament to protest against the measures. The main objection was that the marketisation of services was seen as placing the health visiting service on a par with cleaning and laundry services which had already been privatised. It was, in effect, a fear of deskilling and proletarianisation.

Despite widespread opposition, the government announced its intention to extend fundholding and to place GPs in the position of 'buying in' specific health visiting services. The publication of a Guidance document to fund-holders (NHSME 1992) outlining the measure of 'flexibility' allowed to GPs in the purchasing of health visitor services and the allocation of a 'notional' amount of time (10 per cent) for public health work, did not really allay the fears of the profession (Potrykus 1992).

The emphasis on the pricing and purchasing of health care services within the internal market raised questions regarding the future of public health in its wider sense, for it was feared that services would only be contracted if they were seen as 'marketable' (Potrykus 1989). Was health visiting marketable?

Already the Well Baby clinics which were the backbone of practice were sited in GP surgeries, and the closure of community clinics was under way. This relocation fundamentally altered the relationship between the health visitor and mothers and children. Health visitors were not the only ones engaged in health promotion, this was increasingly the work of practice nurses in Well Woman clinics, the only remaining specific role was home visiting. The fears and desperation of a declining profession under threat were articulated by the general secretary of the HVA in a widely publicised speech in which she asked 'whither health visiting?' (Goodwin 1988). She argued for health visiting to 're-invent' itself, to work to strictly specified targets and standards, becoming a slimline and new-look service targeting vulnerable groups rather than remaining universalist. The strengths of health visiting were founded upon the close relationship that could be formed between the health visitor and individual families. Visiting the home may have had its problems but it gave the health visitor the opportunity to see for herself the conditions and the surroundings within which people lived their lives. This knowledge was in danger of being lost in the transfer to the GP surgery. At the very moment when policies were formed to place care in the community, the profession with everyday knowledge of the community was being squeezed out.

This was just one of the ironies which beset health policy-makers and professionals in the 1980s and 1990s. Another was that, amid the plans for an efficient and cost effective service, a spectre from an earlier time returned, that of the epidemic.

Aids – a moral discourse of an epidemic

Historians (Altman 1986, Weeks 1989) of the development of the epidemic of Aids (acquired immune deficiency syndrome) and the moral discourse that accompanied it, agree that it was first publicly acknowledged in the USA in 1981.

Aids was at first linked to three main groups; homosexual men, haemophiliacs and, surprisingly, Haitians living mainly in New York, San Francisco and Los Angeles. By 1984, HIV (human immunodeficiency virus) had been identified and named and by then the news of this pandemic had reached Britain and mainland Europe. The moral panic that ensued engulfed the popular press and the media, became a part of right-wing political rhetoric and was to have significance for the structure of health education.

By 1984, the reporting of Aids clearly defined and stigmatised it as a 'gay plague' which as Wellings (1988) records was used just as much by the so-called 'quality' press as by the tabloids. Although the incidence among homosexual men was higher in Europe and the USA than among any other group, this was not the case worldwide. Nevertheless, it was as a gay disease that it became firmly identified and reported by the media. Newspaper reporting of Aids sufferers sought to differentiate between the 'guilty' that is those who 'deserved' it (homosexuals) and the 'innocent' victims (haemophiliacs, babies). The idea that Aids constituted a judgement from God or fate on those who were 'morally degenerate', the framework of what Weeks (1989) has termed the 'new Moralism' formed a discourse which generated ambivalent attitudes towards the funding of research into a cure. The publicised deaths of famous figures such as the film star Rock Hudson, ballet dancer Rudolf Nureyev and pop singer Freddie Mercury further served to point to the decadent nature of the victims and their lifestyles. But projected figures on the rampaging nature of the epidemic and predictions of mass deaths prompted the government to put resources towards Aids support services and research in 1985.

The inadequacy of the health education and public health response to the threat was heavily criticised by among others, Professor Adler, who was Britain's leading Aids expert. The television and cinema campaigns were founded upon images of death and destruction which, given the fact that Aids was defined in the popular mind as solely a 'gay' risk, failed to give correct information to the majority of the population. Following the widespread criticism and advice from the BMA the government distributed the leaflet 'Don't Die of Ignorance' to every household in Britain in 1987. The issue of 'safe sex' now became one of mainstream health education rather than the often hidden and taboo subject it had been previously. Condoms became everyday objects offered for sale in supermarkets, garages, local corner shops and hotel lobbies. This was a fundamental cultural change in Britain, but it also reconstituted the original use of condoms as a means of prevention of sexually transmitted diseases rather than a family planning device. It also redefined the discourse of 'safety' in sex towards a more male perspective (we shall be looking at this cultural change in the next chapter).

But the greatest change came in the direction and organisation which health education about Aids took after the initial impact in the early 1980s, especially among the gay community. In many respects the response to health education aimed at prevention of Aids moved away from the top-down approach of the state-centred health service (Wiseman 1989) and moved to a new model of health education. Self-help and support groups such as the Terrence Higgins Trust, formed in Britain in 1984, were in response to the perceived reluctance of official bodies to fund and really address the issues of an increasingly marginalised 'at risk' population. This new model of self-empowerment, as Homans and Aggleton (1988) have classified it, involved the active participation of members of the gay community and others in a community-orientated model. Organisations such as the Terrence Higgins Trust coordinated services, gave information to health authorities, published guidelines for sexual behaviour and generally raised the profile of action. By 1988, such voluntary organisations had become reliant on state funding to continue their work and in exchange the state was only too happy to hand over responsibility to the new non-professional 'experts'.

This was a new departure. For although voluntary organisations had played a major role in provision of health and social services in the nineteenth and early twentieth centuries, they had always employed professionals to carry out the work. But many projects, such as needle exchanges (Stimson et al. 1989) and drug counselling in the prevention of Aids, now involved non-professionals and even users or previous users themselves. This outreach work among stigmatised and marginalised groups such as intravenous drug users, prostitutes and gays, fell to people working with communities rather than community nurses. The ownership of information and treatment that had been in the hands of the health professionals in all previous epidemics was challenged. Sufferers, carers and others still 'at risk', demanded that their voices be heard. There was a growing refusal to accept the definition given them by the mass media, politicians and the health professional establishment. In the USA especially, groups challenged the clinical trial methodology which was the dominant form in medical research. 'With time ticking away, Aids sufferers voted with their feet, setting up "buyers clubs", making bootleg drugs...or through drug sharing, subverting clinical trials conducted along the classical mould' (Porter 1999:708).

To an extent, the communities took responsibility upon themselves and were enabled to do so because of the stigmatised and feared nature of the disease. In Britain, the gay press increasingly played a part in getting across information which was directly relevant to gays (Mitchell 1999), and at the same time reclaiming an identity which was not one of a passive and morally diseased body.

In 1996, the Health Education Authority transferred the responsibility of all initiatives to the Terrence Higgins Trust. The discourse of Aids is interesting because it signalled a shift in British health service provision and in the identification of defined groups. Community nurses were not prepared or trained to deal with an epidemic of Aids. This epidemic did not, in fact, materialise in Britain despite the projections of the RCN in 1985 that there would be one million cases in Britain by 1990 (Wellings 1988). The inaccuracy of this forecast was fortunate as in 1990 a research study revealed that community nurses felt that they were not confident or experienced enough to deal with Aids cases in the community (Bond et al. 1990). In fact, a quarter of those interviewed felt that they should have the right to refuse to care for Aids patients.

Aids, like cholera in the nineteenth century, had to a degree transformed the way in which epidemics were faced by society. As with cholera, the imposition of quarantine regulations was not feasible, although it operated in a covert way with sanctions against the employment of homosexuals in some occupations. Compulsory universal HIV testing was not adopted although doctors did win a court case in 1999 to test a baby whose HIV positive parents had refused permission. Although the epidemic has not (as yet) reached Britain in the feared proportions, nevertheless, on a worldwide scale the danger is still very real. In 1999, the UN (United Nations) warned that a record number of deaths was expected for the year despite an improvement in survival rates in affluent western societies (BMJ 1999:1387).

Unlike cholera or other similiar epidemics, however, combating Aids did not include social reform of housing or public health regulations, but it did signal a significant cultural shift. Community nursing, despite fears, did not become heavily involved. The hospital treatment of Aids in the early years developed into a medication regime and counselling which was undertaken in specialist clinics and centres. But a lesson of 'self-empowerment' had been learnt. It was shown that a stigmatised group could form a communal identity and take a degree of responsibility, it was a challenge to the authoritarian culture of the time. Community nurses had not been instrumental in the governmentality mechanism over a group who, even if marginalised, were overwhelmingly, male, white, educated and articulate.

Aids was a representation of homosexuality as a challenge to the model of 'the family' which was so much a part of the New Right vocabulary, but so too was child abuse – the other moral panic of the 1980s.

Child protection and the state

The issue of child abuse, and specifically sexual abuse, became one of the great publicised concerns of the 1980s. In many ways, it represented a 're-discovery' in that child abuse had been a recognised 'social problem' since the nineteenth century. As Saraga (1993) chronicles, there have been historical stages in which child abuse has been a focus of political concerns. During the 1960s, the 'battered child syndrome' was appropriated by the medical and health professions to place child neglect and abuse within a medical model. Within this model the child was constituted within the sick role as the 'patient' (Parton 1985) and definitions such as 'failure to thrive' and 'neglect' were used to 'play down' the legal aspects and focus upon the condition as one of possible prevention. Families were labelled as 'at risk' in order to search for a predictor of future abuse and it entered into preventive health and social work practice. But why did the issue of child sexual abuse become such a widespread concern in the 1980s?

Gordon (1989) has argued that child abuse becomes a public issue at times when feminism is in the ascendant and women's issues are given a high profile. But the subject of child abuse, like homosexuality in the Aids debate, also came to be an ideological representation of the breakdown of the family within a right-wing political discourse. This was summed up by a speech in Parliament during a debate on child abuse in 1986, when a Conservative member stated that,

> (the prophets of the permissive society) . . . should now be able to recognise the social wreckage that they have helped to encourage (Braine 1986, quoted in Frost and Stein 1989:48).

Child welfare policy is essentially political in framing and implementation (Frost and Stein 1989). Child abuse was seen as a product of a new type of 'dysfunctional' family structure; that of the single or divorced mother with a succession of live-in boyfriends or, at best, a stepfather in residence. Women, as mothers, were often seen as being to 'blame' for either a failure to 'protect' their child from abuse or as being a willing and freely acting accomplice. Female medical and social work professionals were also singled out for being 'over zealous', 'obsessed man hater' or 'incompetent' in the detection or diagnosis of abuse, as was evidenced by the misogynistic treatment of the female paediatrician and chief social worker in the Cleveland Inquiry in 1987 (Campbell 1988). The moral panic over the incidences of child abuse which dominated the popular press during the 1980s activated two major responses; the new discourse on the recognition of the rights of children and the government emphasis upon inter-agency service provision.

Abuse of children was patently not a recent phenomenon but, as Saraga (1993:47) argues, the 'discourses surrounding it are new and for the first time there is a demand to hear "the voices of the children"'.

But these voices were heard and publicised by a variety of child welfare groups and voluntary organisations. As with Aids it was the 'self-empowerment' movement which prompted much of the high-profile debates and also some subsequent prosecutions. The foundation of the counselling service for children, Childline, was set up in 1986 and was swamped with calls, it was estimated that an average of 10,000 calls were made each day in 1987 (*Daily Telegraph*, 1987 in Frost and Stein 1989:71). The experiences and treatment of children in care are represented by National Association of Young People in Care (NAYIC), which evolved from a small group in Leeds in the 1970s to being a national organisation by the early 1980s. The significance of this organisation is that it is comprised of young people acting for themselves and formulating collective demands of the system. This is even more remarkable when it is remembered that the overwhelming majority of children in care come from poor and deprived backgrounds.

The connection between poverty and 'problem families' and consequent incarceration and institutionalisation is one which dominates any history of child welfare. But response to the defining 'moment' of the 1980s, the Cleveland child abuse scandal, although centring the child as the focus of concern also sidestepped the issue of structural poverty.

The events in Cleveland in the summer of 1987 dominated press and media reporting and prompted a full government and judicial inquiry. The press reports concentrated upon the grievances of the families whose children had been 'removed', upon the supposed motives of the female paediatrician, the inefficiency of the social workers and the crisis of family life (Campbell 1988). The subsequent Inquiry prompted the Children Act of 1989 with its intended focusing upon the primacy of the 'interests of the child'. The change in definition of the child was summed up in the words of the Judge Butler-Sloss when she stated 'the child is a human being not an object of concern' (Butler-Sloss, quoted in Campbell 1988:245).

The main significance of the Butler-Sloss Inquiry for the provision of services and encapsulated in the Children Act was the emphasis upon inter-agency working and a relationship of partnership between health and social services and families. This intention signalled a shift in service provision towards a needs-led service with the emphasis on support of families rather than a policing role for social workers and health visitors (Coulton et al. 1998). Social workers and health visitors were now enjoined to 'work together' and although in many instances new collaborative partnerships did emerge, health visitors, as we have seen, were constrained by their place in the new contract culture of the NHS. Child protection was traditionally one of the primary components of health visiting practice but it was social services that became the lead agency in the move to a 'needs-led' service.

Care in and by the community

Within the political-cultural framework of individualism and the imposition of market values in the health service, the dominant organisational shift during the 1990s was towards community-based care. As we have seen, this was not a new idea, it had been around since the late 1950s and early 1960s. But it was during this period that the ideal of 'community' became an organising principle of replacing a reliance on professional and formal care with one of care *by* the community. From 1985 onwards, a series of reports and White Papers advocated a move to a more fragmented and mixed economy of care provision that placed the main responsibility for care on to the community. But exactly who in the 'community' was to be the main provider? Many writers have pointed to the essential ambiguity of the concept of 'community' (Titmus 1979, Williams 1983, Skidmore 1994, 1997, Symonds and Kelly 1998). But it is this ambiguity that allows for its strength as a means of denoting a site and responsibility for health and social care. Within the 'new' health service the main responsibility for the provision of health and social care was removed from the state and placed within a set of contractual relationships with the voluntary sector, the market and individual families and friends. The role of the state changed from that of provider to that of an 'enabler' or purchaser.

Within the NHS and Community Care Act of 1990, which was implemented in 1992, the distinction between health and social care was made with the responsibility being 'split' between the health service and social services with the latter as the lead agency. Social services departments were required to annually produce projected Care Plans for the area and to contract out specific services to voluntary organisations as well as some private organisations. This resulted in a larger role for the voluntary sector, but as Leat (1995) has shown, this was not without its problems. The voluntary sector was placed in a contradictory position, involved with the market and yet outside, relying on volunteers and yet required to bid for contracts in a professional way as a service provider for an enabling state (Drake 1998).

The formal distinction made between health and social care, which was coupled with the expressed encouragement for a closer collaboration between agencies and professions, distinguished the work of community nurses, social workers and care workers for voluntary and private organisations. Furthermore, under the Act, health care and nursing provision remained within the health service and free at the point of need, whereas designated social care was to be means-tested.

Within the new and narrow managerialist culture of the health service, this was interpreted as a means by which the actual practice of district nurses was scrutinised and classified according to the 'skill' required to perform clinical assessment, health care or social care tasks. The organisation of district nurses into 'skill-mix' teams, was undertaken in order to rationalise and demarcate duties and tasks. The generic and all-encompassing role of district nursing as envisaged by Florence Nightingale and others a century before, was replaced by a fragmented and targeted service which was shared with many grades and variously qualified workers.

But *who* in the community were considered to be the most suitable recipients of care? Ironically, it was primarily the two groups who had always been so defined; the frail elderly and the mentally ill. We have to make a distinction here between the responsibility to 'care' that was applied to both these groups, and the responsibility to 'protect' which was applied to children and involved health visitors and social workers. The responsibility to care for the long-term sick and frail elderly and those with a mental illness was shared by district nurses, other care workers, and community psychiatric nurses and social workers.

The informal care given by families, relatives and friends increasingly became a recognised part of the system of community-based care. The politicisation of carers into a recognised 'movement' and a growing body of sociological research into caring (Finch and Groves 1983, Dalley 1988, Ungerson 1987) brought this hitherto hidden area of predominantly unpaid female care into the spotlight (Bytheway and Johnson 1998). The involvement and consultation between social workers and carers over the packages of care to be received was a requirement of the Community Care Act, and this further devolved responsibility from the nursing professionals.

Although the numbers of elderly people being cared for in the community was by far the largest in terms of numbers, it was the minority of mental health patients who attracted widespread publicity and fuelled a moral panic over the 'mad on the streets'.

The 'failure' of community care

The process of 'de-hospitalisation' that began in the early 1980s was destined to be highly controversial. The image of the 'mad on the streets' emerging from the shadows and evoking a picture of Victorian menace is a powerful one which has become almost synonomous in the media with 'community care' (Wilkinson 1998). The 1990s saw a series of sensationalised events such as the picture of a self-discharged psychiatric patient, Ben Silcock, captured on a TV camera climbing the bars of a lions' enclosure in London Zoo in 1991, which was transmitted on all the evening news programmes. The catalogue of horrific deaths of both the patients and 'innocent' victims as well as TV documentaries illustrating the shortage of psychiatric beds in hospitals continued to dominate any reference to community care throughout the 1990s.

In a report on increased violence in Accident and Emergency units, a description of the overpowering of a man by police, nurses and doctors in such an incident it was stated:

> The nurses are in broad agreement about the circumstances that have fostered the increase in such incidents. Care in the community, they say, has been a disaster, leading to hugely raised numbers of violently disturbed people on the streets. (*The Independent* 1999:R1)

In the same week, there was a violent incident in a church service in London when a naked man waving a sword badly injured many in the congregation. Incidents such as these and the resultant public anxiety was addressed by changes in policy. In 1994, the then Secretary of State for Health, Virginia Bottomley, announced changes to the legislation after admitting that in the policy implementation of community care for mental health paients 'the pendulum had swung too far' (Audit Commission 1994). The change was to introduce an amendment to the 1983 Mental Health Act (Mental Health (Patients in the Community) Act 1995) in which a system of supervision orders were to be issued to a named key worker who would supervise the patients and their treatment. This key worker was nearly always a community psychiatric nurse.

The process of 'de-hospitalisation' affected not only the patients, but the organisation and structure of mental health nursing. The organisation of community psychiatric nursing had undergone great change during this period, 'the primary obligation in the future would be to community mental health teams' (Shears and Coleman 1999:1386). But of course the training of new entrants and the lifetime experience of others was based in the setting of the hospital or institution. The position was further complicated by the structure of the new health service. The thrust of government concern was that mental health teams in the community would target the care of the seriously mentally ill, but the advent of GP fundholding in 1991 meant that GPs purchased mental health care provision for their patients. As Shears and Coleman (1999) argue, the two agencies did not coincide. GPs tended to refer to the community psychiatric nurse (CPN) the less seriously mentally ill cases which were by far the more numerous, predominantly cases of post-natal depression and anxiety counselling. White (1993) published a study of community psychiatric nursing which showed that only one in five people suffering from schizophrenia were on a CPN caseload, a situation described by Gournay (1994) as 'scandalous'. By 1995, the situation prompted a call by some inner city trust executives for a large investment of 50 million to build up urban services for the seriously mentally ill (*Health Service Journal* 1995:26). In this report, it was calculated that the cost of lifetime care for a person with severe mental illness such as schizophrenia could be as much as £700,000 per patient. Faced with this sort of cost, the New Labour government in 1997 decided upon another option, a return to a revised form of institutionalised care.

Communitarianism – a new political discourse

As we shall see in Chapter 3, there was a recognition by the latter years of the 1990s that the certainties which had underpinned British society were rapidly disintegrating. The 'ideal' nuclear family was in retreat, divorce rates and single parenthood were increasing, juvenile unemployment and crime was a constant concern, parts of large cities had become virtual 'no-go' areas, and economic and social decline was also affecting rural areas. In many ways, certain localities and social problems would have been instantly recognisable to nineteenth-century reformers. It was against this background that the New Labour government achieved a landslide victory in 1997. As with the election of the New Right in 1979, the radically different nature of New Labour policies compared to the ones pursued by previous Labour administrations was not at first perceived. Nevertheless, it soon became obvious that a new political and ideological formation was in place and not just a continuation of traditional Labour policies. What constituted this new approach?

One of the intellectual supporters of this new approach, Anthony Giddens (1994), coined the phrase 'the Third Way' to describe the political placement of policy direction. This phrase was increasingly used to describe an alternative to both the reliance on state welfarism of the early postwar period and the imposition of market values which followed during the 1980s and 1990s. This new direction signalled an emphasis on community regeneration, social inclusion and cohesiveness rather than either a state paternalism or market individualism. We would argue that like the previous two periods of welfare provision this present phase is also based upon a conception of the human body. The period of social efficiency which was replaced by an emphasis on the individual body is being superceded by the concept of the community as a body. The state under this political-cultural project is to engage in social investment in education and health but is not to return to being the sole provider of welfare. The 'mixed economy' is to remain with a role for both the private and voluntary sectors. The concept of inclusion is a very important one, with the ideal of a 'cosmopolitan nation' which will replace a 'conservative nation' (Giddens 1998).

Another supporter of the new discourse, Le Grand, summed up the philosophy of the new Third Way under the acronym CORA – community, opportunity, responsibility and accountability (Le Grand 1998:26). This framework embodies a belief in community as a value and a site. The process of devolution for Scotland and Wales and a separate administration for London, coupled with increased powers for local authorities and organisations were indicative of this communitarian belief. The rights of individuals as parents and workers were to be strengthened but so too was their responsibility. Parents were to be made more legally responsible for the public actions and behaviour of children and this responsibility was extended to people as tenants, car owners and patients. The state was to provide the opportunity for people to take up education and training aimed at employment and was also to provide a system of public and state-funded childcare. A National Childcare Strategy was introduced which increased child benefits, gave childcare allowances to mothers wishing to take up work, increased parental leave and initiated many projects aimed at early intervention to prevent the generation of social exclusion. We will be studying the effect of these in Chapter 6.

The public services were to be made accountable. This meant that educational establishments, hospitals and health authorities had to operate within nationally set 'performance frameworks'. Performance indicators were to be set which would monitor the efficiency of all hospitals, medical and nursing services. The objective of constructing this inclusive society was the basis of establishing the Social Exclusion Unit in 1997. This unit, within the Cabinet and reporting directly to the Prime Minister, was required to report back on measures on 'tackling poverty and social exclusion' (DSS 1999). We will be looking in more depth at the contested notion of this phrase in the following chapter. Nevertheless, with a government committed to both social inclusion and efficiency and 'best value' in the provision of health and social welfare, the political map had changed once more. How were these changes and commitments to affect the delivery of health and community-based services?

New directions and traditional roles

The election of the New Labour government in 1997 heralded another major upheaval in the organisation of the NHS. Initially focused upon a modest and practical aim to reduce waiting lists for hospital treatment, the New Labour discourse on health was to form a major part of the new political-cultural map.

The first upheaval was the abolition of the system of GP fundholding and its replacement by commissioning of health services by local groups consisting of GPs, community nurses, local authority representatives and members of voluntary and patient organisations. The pattern for the new NHS was set out in a series of White Papers for England, Wales and Scotland in 1997.

Another radical break with the past was the appointment of a Minister for Public Health and the publication of reports on the causes and recommendations for the solution to the recognised inequalities in health known as the Acheson Report (DoH 1998a). For the first time, the effect of poverty and deprivation on health was officially recognised by the government. In 2002, the government set targets for the elimination of health inequalities in the NHS Plan, this is discussed in more detail in the following section. However, during the late 1990s, the issue of community care was one that tended to be marginalised amid plans for hospital services, Health Action Zones, and health improvement projects. There was one exception to this, the controversial issue of the community treatment of mental illness. In 1998, the then Secretary of State for Health, Frank Dobson, in his introduction to the White Paper stated that:

> Care in the community has failed because, while it improved the treatment of many people who were mentally ill, it left far too many walking the streets, often at risk to themselves and a nuisance to others. A small but significant minority have been a threat to others or themselves. (DoH 1998b:6)

This report promised a series of measures to strengthen mental health legislation including better outreach services, more secure provision in smaller units, and additional investment to employ up to 15,000 more nurses especially in the mental health services.

Despite this initiative, concern still remained and further publicised cases prompted even more reforms in 1999 announced by the new Health Minister, Alan Milburn who stated that:

> The current mental health laws have failed. They have failed to properly protect the public, patients or staff. The tragic toll of suicides and homicides graphically illustrates the failure. (quoted in BMJ 1999:1389)

The following proposals were for an extension of compulsory treatment in hospital or the community (DoH 1999). Although broadly welcomed by the Royal College of Psychiatrists, the element of compulsion in these proposals attracted opposition from some voluntary groups and the RCN. Importantly however, this Green Paper also signalled a move away from the more laissez-faire approach and a return to the concept of incarceration and the removal from the public gaze of those who were placed outside of society.

On the other hand, childcare which had previously existed in the private sphere of the family home was brought into the public gaze. This move was to have a significant impact upon the declining profession of health visiting.

In 1997, the Health Visitors' Association had changed its name to that of the Community Practitioners and Health Visitors' Association in recognition of the more community nurse-orientated direction in which it was being pushed by some within the profession. However, the new childcare strategy and the emergence of family policies after 1997, effectively re-formulated the health visiting role and its place in public health.

The new political orientation towards the importance of work and of community and parental responsibility specifically designated health visitors as having a pivotal role in the new governmentality. A White Paper published in 1999 clearly set out a new 'enhanced role for health visitors' (Home Office 1998:1.26–1.30). This was part of the government initiative to encourage responsible parenting, to help families 'balance work and family', and also to be a supportive mechanism in the reconstruction of family and community networks. A programme of Sure Start projects, involving partnership with many other agencies, which targets families in socially deprived areas and offers early intervention in the form of advice, counselling and practical help in parenting received government funding and began to be implemented. The high profile given to families and parenting obviously involved a greater role for health visitors in what could be described as a return to their traditional roots in public health. The Sure Start initiatives are discussed in Chapter 6.

School nursing was also to be removed from the margins and given a more centralised role in the new policies. The report by the Social Exclusion Unit on Teenage Pregnancy (SEU 1999a), recommended that school nurses or an 'on site health professional' (SEU 1999a:Annex 4), be responsible for giving contraceptive advice and counselling on sexual behaviour to young people under the age of 16. This recommendation is very reminiscent of that offered in 1943 in the Report on 'problem families' (Womens Group on Public Welfare 1943).

The long-term care of older people was the subject of a Royal Commission set up in 1997 to address the problem of the funding arrangements for the mid and long term. The resultant recommendation was for the extension of joint funding and partnership and cooperation between health and social services (DoH 1998c). The implementation of joint funding for health and social care presents a new and potentially different way of working for community nurses. Although all designated nursing care whether in a residential setting or at home remains free the strategy of skill-mix and team nursing continues. The role of district nursing has changed radically with the most highly qualified taking responsibility for assessment and the construction and management of care plans but with an army of less qualified staff performing the hands-on work. The mixture of health and social care which characterised the traditional nursing role in the community is now compartmentalised. Although health visiting and school nursing services are being placed in the spotlight by new policy directions, the future of psychiatric nursing is more controversial and that of district nursing although fundamental to any community-based care provision is still marginalised by policies. These changes in the organisational structure of community-based nursing, have led to a questioning of the identity of community nursing itself. This debate is undertaken in Chapter 4.

Modernising community services?

The dominant discourse that underpins all current policies is essentially that of *pragmatism*. This is accompanied by the discourse of *modernisation*. How can we identify these two discourses in current policy direction? Pragmatism is summed up in the phrase 'what counts is what works', this in effect has replaced a vision of an ideal system. An ideological commitment to a specific political philosophy which underpinned the foundation of the NHS in 1948, and also the market reforms of the 1980s, has been replaced by a managerialist ethos which lays stress on the delivery of results. But the pragmatic approach which focuses upon the achievement of results must of necessity have in place a set of bench-marks or standards of 'best practice' to which service providers must conform. The current emphasis on targets, audits and continuous evaluation are all means by which 'what works' can be assessed. Modernisation in this context has come to be identified with the application of sets of targets and measurable outcomes to the provision of health and social care. The existence of many different partners in the provision of care has rendered it essential that the old, taken-for-granted assumptions of achievement be standardised and systematically structured.

After 2001, the second New Labour administration sought to address the perceived problems of the NHS which were popularly defined as; inadequate funding, inefficiency and inequalities of service provision. A large injection of money is promised in order to raise health spending in Britain to that of the average investment in Europe, the projected target was 9.4 per cent of GDP (gross domestic product) by 2008. Although it is primarily hospital services that are the focus of targets of health service provision and of publicised concerns, nevertheless, community care services are included in new policies.

The NHS Plan and the strategies for delivery (DoH 2002) are based upon the recognition that 'the 1948 model is simply inadequate for today's needs' (DoH 2002:1). The method of funding the NHS through taxation is to remain but the supply of services is to be transformed from a state monopoly to a diversity of suppliers. The involvement of private finance in the NHS is, at present, a controversial issue, but the expansion of partnership working between the statutory services, the health service, social services and the voluntary sector is a requisite. The plurality of provision is in contrast to the state monopoly of provision that characterised the postwar welfare state.

The basic tenet of care being provided 'free at the point of need' has also been affected by the new regulations regarding the care provided to frail older people. As we have seen, the recommendations made by the Royal Commission on the Long-Term Care for the Elderly (DoH 1999) set patterns for skill-mix within community nursing practice. But the most controversial issue to emerge from this report is the question of the costs of personal care as opposed to defined nursing care to be delivered to individuals. The main body of the Commission recommended that personal care, defined as those tasks which though essential to physical and mental wellbeing did not require the services of a professional nurse, be free of charge. However, it was the minority report that recommended that payment for personal care be means tested that has become government policy in England and Wales. This policy has attracted opposition from many quarters and the Scottish Parliament has opted to provide personal care free of charge. What is interesting, however, is the formalised division between 'nursing' and 'personal' care which is now accepted but which would have been inexplicable to previous generations of community nurses.

The focus upon partnership working between the statutory sectors of health and social services is illustrated by the policy changes regarding the financial responsibilities for care of older people. Under the NHS Plan, local authorities are made responsible for the costs of hospital 'bed blocking' by older people. Social services will be required to use their funds to provide a range of home care services. NHS hospitals are to be made financially responsible for the cost of emergency re-admissions.

The diversity of provision of care services has led to a need for providers to be accountable for quality and standards of care. The Care Standards Act 2000 established a National Care Standards Commission for the regulation of many sites of public care including; children's homes, care homes, domiciliary care agencies and nurse agencies. Importantly, it also made provision for the regulation and inspection of voluntary adoption agencies as well as local authority fostering and adoption services. The training and regulation of social care workers is undertaken by the General Social Care Council in England, and the Care Council for Wales. In Wales, a Children's Commissioner has been appointed to oversee the protection of looked-after children. The public care of children is now focused upon by the Children's Safeguard Review set up in response to the publicising of the perpetuation of child abuse in residential children's homes in recent years.

In addition to the setting of standards of quality of care, one of the major organisational changes to the provision of community services is the implementation of targets to be achieved in respect of the tackling of health inequalities and community regeneration. The concepts of active citizenship and social inclusion are now seen as the primary objective of policies and community nurses are required to be involved in what was previously defined as community development. We will pursue this point in the following chapter.

Summary

In this chapter it has been argued that there have been three distinct political-cultural discourses in the years from 1940 until the present. The first, which saw the foundation of the NHS in 1948, set the pattern for the hospital domination of the structure and organisation of health care. But this was enacted within the framework of a political culture that saw free and universal access to medical expertise as the defining element of a social democracy. The war years promoted a vision of social cohesion and equality that was set in stark contrast to the economic and social deprivation that had characterised the immediate pre-war years. The provision of health to all citizens was an accepted responsibility of government and the main concern was that of the 'social efficiency' of the body of the population. But this entailed a distinctive definition of health and health care that was unambiguously that of the medical model and, as such, established the dominance of the medical profession in the NHS. Although this undoubtedly paid dividends in the sense that the population as a whole enjoyed a longer expectation of life, infectious diseases were controlled, infant and maternal mortality declined, for the first time in history, the idea of an 'ageing' population presented a social problem. The improvement in the social efficiency and health of the body of the British population had been achieved, but at a cost. The overwhelming belief in the welfare state as a mechanism for ensuring 'cradle to grave' support and security appeared inviolable in the decades following the end of the war.

After three decades of increased prosperity and affluence, however, by the late 1970s, the question of whether this welfare could be afforded began to be asked. The concerns over cost, increasing unemployment and inflation, the growing divisions in society, all coalesced in the moves from the margins of an alternative political-cultural discourse.

The construction of a social and economic philosophy which emphasised the role of the individual rather than the collective, of profit not service and of competition rather than cooperation was the response to these concerns. Within this discourse, health became a consumer good which could be gained by personal endeavour and responsibility. The body of the individual was now the focus of policies that set targets for health gain, emphasised healthy behaviour, and reorganised the health service as a 'quasi-market'. The value of competition between doctors, hospitals and other agencies was the spur to an increased efficiency of delivery of health care within a managerialist culture. The individual body was that of a consumer of health care engaged in a search for the best bargain. Ironically, this move tended to demystify the concept of health and redefine it as a product that was manufactured and exchanged within a market. This move rendered the structural inequalities inherent in markets visible and obvious. The growing divide in the health of the nation between rich and poor, men and women, ethnic groups, young and old, became the subject of reports. By the early 1990s, the social and economic divisions within Britain resembled those of a century before.

Against this background, another political-cultural discourse was framed. The emphasis now turned to social inclusion and a regeneration of communities. The social body and the individual body were now replaced by the body of the community. The route to social inclusion of the no-go areas and the visible underclass lay with work and family responsibility. This new philosophy which combined a traditional work ethic with a new emphasis on personal achievement also constructed a community body which was (like the representative human body of the Millenium Dome) gender-less, class-less and opaque. Health was defined as a right of citizenship and a personal responsibility.

Within these changing discourses, the role and organisation of community nursing has constantly been redefined and reformed. The organisation and role of all branches of community nursing and health visiting have reflected the changes in political-cultural discourses. Community nursing became a part of the welfare state in the postwar period and was then subjected to the quasi-market practice of contract during the 1980s and early 1990s. At present, under current policy direction, new enhanced roles for health visiting and school nursing are envisaged but the tasks of district nursing and mental nursing are undergoing change.

Community nursing has always been the public face of nursing. Although organisations and roles may have changed, it is community nurses whom most people actually see on a daily basis. Unlike hospital nurses, they are a part of the landscape of 'normal' life, public and approachable. They are present in shops, in the street and in peoples' homes.

Despite the fact that issues of public health, primary health care and community-based services have received a high profile in current government policies, hospital services still dominate the politics of health care. All nurses are trained initially in hospitals and are immersed in an institutional culture which has to be 'unlearned' when transferring to community nursing. Although partnerships with other agencies, especially the social services, are frequently emphasised, the two are often working and training in totally different cultures.

In these first two chapters the construction of branches of community nursing has been traced through the various and often competing discourses which have formed the cultural maps of the time.

We now turn to look at the community settings within which community nurses are placed and where they construct their practice.

CHAPTER 3

Constructing Communities: Policies and Cultures

Introduction

This chapter focuses upon two main issues; the siting and construction of communities by social policies and the subsequent significance of the discourse of 'community' to the making of social policies. It will be argued that this is very much a two-way process, policies construct visible and definable 'communities' and in turn the concept and discourse of 'community' is embedded in current social policies.

The previous two chapters have reviewed the historical development of community nursing, this chapter focuses upon the construction of the everyday reality of the site of practice. This discourse and the policies that are, at present, being founded upon a definition of community and social cohesion are of great importance to the practice and future of community nursing and this will be discussed in depth in Chapter 4. It is important that the link between the setting and the reconstruction of the role of community nursing be recognised. This changing role and its relationship to the changing nature of communities is discussed in depth in Chapter 5. In Chapter 6, we look at the current policy directions in tackling the problems that are seen as an outcome of a 'decline' in traditional community life. Community nurses are being brought into the mechanism of governmentality by policies that are targeting groups and areas of social exclusion. In order to understand this process we must place it within a historical and social context.

Definitions of 'community' are very difficult to conclusively pin down, but in this chapter there will be two main definitions in use; firstly, the application of 'community' to an area or locality and secondly, the use of 'community' to denote a social or cultural identity. In some instances, a social identity, for example 'working class' is attached to a specific locality. Ethnic identities too are applied to localities, an 'Asian area', or an 'Irish area', and the designation of certain areas as 'no-go' or 'problem estates'. But it must be remembered that these areas were constructed by specific policies as well as changing social and economic conditions. Places *become* 'problem estates', 'deprived areas' or 'racially-mixed' through external structural conditions and rarely by intent. Over time people living in certain areas construct a social reality that is essentially a response to historical conditions and present circumstances. Certain areas develop and construct 'cultures' whether it is the middle-class culture of the residential suburbs, the street culture of traditional working-class areas, or the seemingly anarchic or tribal culture of the problem estates. These sub-cultures are also divided by factors of gender, ethnicity and age. Therefore, to accurately construct a community profile is a very complex task involving history, economic structures, knowledge of criss-crossing cultures and norms of behaviour as well as empirical data on population, income, health statistics and demographic change. In this chapter, we will look at the construction of localities through housing and other social policies. It will be argued that these localities then take on a social identity and reality. We will focus upon; changing definitions of social class and locality, of ethnicity, age and gender and their relationship to localities constructed by social policies. We will also look in more depth at 'communities' which are outside of a permanent locality and of mainstream society; for example, the homeless street people. The second part of the process, the construction of social policies upon a discourse of community itself will involve a study of contemporary issues and concerns. The phrase social exclusion and its corollary, social inclusion, dominate British social policies of the present. In many ways, this is reminiscent of the late nineteenth-century concerns over the management of the poor and the 'unfit' section of the population. There are, however, differences in both approach and social definitions that reflect a changed culture and view of the world. Current policies, although aimed at social cohesion and the elimination of exclusion are not circumscribed by the maintenance of traditional structures of class, gender or race. Societal divisions remain but they are of a different nature and composition. For example, the new welfarism is not based upon the male breadwinner but upon the figure of the universal worker. High priority is given to 'parenting' and not 'motherhood' and the distinction between the public sphere of work and the private sphere of the family is becoming blurred. Health is a very much wider concept than in the past, and involves not just the absence of disease but the reduction of risk and the personal responsibility of the individual underpinned by the public duty of the state. The new policy direction of inclusion necessitates the mechanism of governmentality and it is to community nurses that much of this responsibility is being addressed. Before we look at the construction of communities, however, it would be useful to unpack the social meaning that has become attached to the phrase 'community'.

Community and cultures

Many writers have pointed to the *ideological* significance of the concept of community. The 'dream world' of a community was defined by Williams as being one of the 'key words' in our culture (Williams 1983). It is this dream world of a community in which all 'belong' and have a defined identity and role which is the basis of the familiar soap operas which are followed by millions in Britain and throughout the industrialised world. Sociologically, it could be argued that as societies have become more fragmented and people more isolated, so a desire to 'be where everyone knows your name' grows stronger.

This dream community that existed in some indeterminate past may have an existence in the imagination but often does not bear close scrutiny or analysis. Even personal reminiscences of long-lost communities reveal that there were always marginalised individuals or groups who were excluded on grounds of race, respectability or 'strangeness' (Symonds and Kelly 1998:13). During the initial moves towards the implementation of a policy of community-based care, the social policy theorist Richard Titmus warned of the danger of confusing the cultural identity of community 'the everlasting cottage garden' with an often harsh social reality (Titmus 1979). Among recent writings of the meaning of community is the argument by Chen (1999) that the need for a re-theorising of the meaning of community has arisen due to the social and economic changes that have occurred since the inception of the postwar welfare state.

In the heyday of social democracy, the notion of 'community' needed little theorising. British society was constructed around communities – local communities, trade-based and industrial ones and the larger collectivities of class. Most people's outlook on life, and certainly on politics was coloured by these social identities Chen (1999:13).

These communities now in decline are defined as *ascribed*, meaning that they were externally constructed and lacked any element of individual choice. This is contrasted with a new type of collectivity, that of *elective* communities which are bound together by lifestyle, interests and identities and are self-chosen. We would add a third dimension to this typology, that of *marginalised* communities who exist on the very periphery of society. Figure 3.1 demonstrates this typology of communities and their characteristics.

There are complexities which can be added to this model, for example a previously ascribed community can change to an elective or a marginalised one. An instance of this would be an area such as Brixton which may have been ascribed to the first Afro-Caribbean immigrants to Britain in the 1950s, but now may well be where many of a later generation even though they have acquired a better socio-economic status have chosen to reside because of the network of relationships, interests and feeling of belonging. Areas such as this, of course, offer a measure of security and solidarity to people who may experience the impact of racism in areas that are predominantly white. This has led in some areas to exclusively black or Asian and 'poor white' areas of residence. This segregation led in the summer of 2001 to violent confrontations in northern cities such as Blackburn. In the same way, previously ascribed areas which were based upon one industry such as the mining areas of South Wales and the North of England have now disintegrated into semi-marginal ones where structural unemployment has produced a panoply of social problems.

Figure 3.1 A typology of 'ideal type' communities

Ascribed	Elective	Marginalised
Class-based Production role	Income-based Consumption role	Existence
Uniform	Diverse	Uniform
Role specific	Role diverse	Role specific
Geographically-centred locality networks	Cultural networks	Locality of shared need
Externally constructed	Voluntaristic	Externally constructed Individual response
Occupation based	Lifestyle	Uniformity of marginality
Civic/individualised culture	Civic/group culture	Individualised/deviant culture

A degree of fluidity has to be recognised when attempting to clearly define 'ideal types' of communities. Within one identifying characteristic, minority ethnic groups or rural communities, for instance, many divisions within the groups can be seen. As we shall discuss later in this chapter, communities and localities can be both elective and ascribed and even marginalised at the same time.

The concept of community in recent years has become attached to a notion of citizenship. Both denote a relationship between the individual and the larger structures of locality or state, a sense of belonging. In the social-democratic settlement of the postwar years, the definition of citizenship was constructed as a set of political, social and economic 'rights' (Marshall 1950), namely: the right to vote and to stand for election, the right to employment and equality of justice before the law. Although these rights were always more applicable to working men rather than home-based women and to the ethnic majority rather than minorities, to the physically and mentally able rather than those with a disability – nevertheless, they served as a sort of benchmark of citizenship. After the social upheavals of the 1980s and 1990s, a new concept entered into the political vocabulary, that of social exclusion. This phrase which has become popular currency and upon which the Social Exclusion Unit (SEU) was formed in 1998, is one that is new to the British context. What does it mean? The actual indices of social exclusion are ambiguous, poverty is of course the primary ingredient but not the only one. It incorporates educational failure, long-term unemployment, single state-supported motherhood, dependency on means-tested benefits and on the unregulated black economy. But as well as its application to *individual* characteristics, it also encompasses *localities* where whole communities share some or all of these individualised

Figure 3.2   Cultures of social exclusion/inclusion

Civic culture – social inclusion	*Individualised culture of social exclusion*
Secure employment/retirement Educationally aware Financially confident	Long-term unemployment/state supported Educational failure Long-term poverty
Responsible families/relationships High mobility/access to private/public transport	Families with problems Low mobility/limited access to public transport
Participation in civic activities: voting, volunteering, caring/membership of clubs or societies/public office	Isolated/participation in deviant or criminal activities
Outward directed/inclusive	Inward directed/exclusive
Predominant group in ascribed and elective communities	**Entire or section of ascribed communities** **Marginalised communites**

disadvantages. It also illustrates a conceptual move from the focus upon the individual to one on the *community* as a whole. This communitarianism is, we would argue, the motivating force behind current social policies. However, before looking at the direction of policies, a view of the *culture* that underpins the different types of communities is indicative of their potential for social exclusion/inclusion. As Figure 3.2 illustrates, as well as structural characteristics communities can possess *cultural* ones. The possession of a civic culture, we would argue, is a prerequisite for social inclusion.

Again a caveat must be added to this model, a civic culture may not be adhered to by everybody in a community but if it is the dominant one then it will be isolated individuals or families which will be socially excluded. This can often be the case in farming and agricultural areas. Equally, certain individuals living in largely socially excluded communities on, for instance, a 'no-go' estate, may attempt to develop or retain a more outward-looking culture of civic responsibility. These individuals often attempt to organise tenants' associations or community projects and are frequently seen by outside professionals as community leaders or representatives of the 'decent' minority.

It is not feasible therefore to simply 'read off' a culture from a locality, this would be far too simplistic. But both dominant and peripheral cultures that may co-exist must be taken into account when a community is being profiled.

People create a culture over time as a response to pre-existing conditions and circumstances. The construction of ascribed communities on the basis of social class was undertaken by state policies within a specific historical and economic context. The secure postwar communities which underpinned the welfare state were as much a construction of policies as their decline into marginalised 'problem estates' in the 1980s.

Cultural divisions within what may be loosely termed the working class are deep and have historically been seen as indications of difference and fragmentation. The division between the 'respectable' and the 'rough' working class has a long tradition and there is an extensive list of definitions of the section of the poor who were always seen as existing outside of mainstream working-class life and of social citizenship (Morris 1994). There are many other social and economic gradations that have existed since industrialisation, based upon regional differences, between rural and urban areas, religious affiliations and occupations. Communities were always more than just localities within which people lived and worked, they were also cultural sites of identity. Housing policies throughout the nineteenth and twentieth centuries have both built upon, reinforced and constructed cultural divisions. The provision of housing for working-class people represented a social and economic problem, one that was initially placed with the market and then with the state. But it was through the attempted resolution of this problem that working-class-ascribed communities came into being.

Social divisions and housing reform

Booth's study of poverty in London in the 1880s (Booth 1902) vividly described the social divisions within the broad spectrum of the working class. In this study, it was calculated that nearly a third (30.7 per cent) of the population were living in poverty. This number included the working poor as well as the 'residium' which was calculated to be approximately 10 per cent of the population. Although this large proportion of people had poverty in common, it was the moral degeneracy of the lowest stratum which set them apart. As Keating has noted, the residium were regarded as 'unrescuable'; 'Occasional labourers, street-sellers, loafers, criminals and semi-criminals . . . They degrade whatever they touch and as individuals are incapable of improvement' (Keating 1976:114).

The distinction between this group and the labouring poor, reliant on casual work and existing on the brink of starvation, as identified by Booth in his studies, was ambiguous to outside observers, but probably very real to those struggling to create an identity of respectability. The necessity to distinguish themselves from the lowest stratum is a theme which runs through much historical autobiography:

> outside my little world of gas-lighted bedrooms, the kitchen with the blazing coal
> fire, the parlour which was seldom used, with its creaking floor boards that set the
> china on the dresser jingling...there was the street outside, where children played
> round lamp posts, where the lamp lighter came with lighted pole each evening....
> but beyond that corner my world ended. Away down the road were the cluttered
> streets of dockland, with pubs on the corners, where barefoot children begged for
> half pennies. My father's £2 a week was adequate to screen me from such poverty.
> (Burnett 1982:27)

Until the latter decades of the nineteenth century, the respectable working
class, such as the family of this writer, lived in close proximity to the disreputable poor. But yet another division within the working class had been created by industrial and technological advance. The historical creation of the
'labour aristocracy', the skilled and relatively well-paid section of the working
class, began to make social advancement by the latter decades of the nineteenth century (Hobsbawm 1968, Foster 1974). This group undeniably had
the economic power to exercise a measure of control over their life chances in
the labour market (Mann 1992). These were the (men) who were the founders
of the Cooperative movement, who started savings clubs and contributed to
insurance schemes, and who formed the membership of the new model trade
unions. Many of this class now had the vote and formed a constituency with
political power. They also had created welfare provision for themselves and
were not reliant on the Poor Law for subsistence in times of hardship and were
relatively safe from pauperism. This relatively affluent and influential section
of the working class gained cultural power.

> This distinctiveness of this upper stratum of the working class is not that its
> members joined thrift and voluntary institutions, for so to an extent did lesser skilled
> and unskilled workers. The real point is that they joined so many that at one level it
> materially affected their life chances and experiences...while at another level...it
> helped determine their values and their culture. (Crossick 1978:132)

The divisions within the working class were based not only on wage differentials but upon the *cultures* which identified each strata. The burgeoning civic
culture of the upper stratum and other groups of the aspiring respectable
working poor was in stark contrast to the unregulated street life based upon
begging and petty crime which was indicative of the 'residium'.

The housing conditions of the groups within the lower strata of the working class differed, but it was the existence of the overcrowded city slums that
gave the most concern to public health officials. The public nature of the
extreme poverty and destitution visible from the streets was recorded by early
photographers and was given publicity by the growing popular press.

The housing conditions of the poor in the malodorous and overcrowded urban slums of the nineteenth century were the subject of much political concern at the time (Stedman-Jones 1971, Gaudie 1974). The basis of this concern was the prevention and containment of epidemics. The direct result of the focus on the overcrowded slums as the cause of disease was not to increase housing provision.

> The need to curb epidemics became urgent and so the removal of filth caused by overcrowding became the reformers' goal, leaving overcrowding itself not only untreated but increasing...The provision of more houses was not pressed. Instead of being treated as a subject in its own right, housing became one part and a neglected part, of the public health campaign. (Gaudie 1974:85)

The provision of housing for the working class was initially undertaken by philanthropic organisations in the mid nineteenth century. Some of these organisations such as the Peabody Trust actually built blocks of flats for working-class families many of whom had been displaced by the wholesale demolition of areas by the new Railway Companies in London. Rooms in these buildings were available at a reasonable rent to the 'respectable' working class and there were numerous rules concerning the conduct and personal behaviour of the tenants. Many of the working class resented these restrictions and nicknamed the buildings 'Bastilles'.

Other housing reformers such as Octavia Hill focused upon the renovation and maintenance of existing properties and rented them to families in exchange for cooperation and a degree of self-help. The underlying agenda in these philanthropic projects was not just to provide housing but to engage in social engineering.

Octavia Hill personified the Victorian desire for reform of the poor and the need for the management of poverty. From the 1860s, she employed 'lady collectors and visitors' who went among the poor not just collecting the rents but ensuring that standards of cleanliness and hygiene were upheld. Octavia Hill was adamant that, for the very poor, housing could never be provided at a market rent. Her tenants belonged to what she herself called 'the destructive classes' (Ravetz 1989:191), and she therefore concentrated on the reform of the tenants rather than buildings. Another form of housing provision throughout the latter part of the nineteenth century, was that of the 'model' villages which were constructed by large employers for their workers. These schemes, at their best, represented a new and radical vision of working-class housing.

Places such as Bourneville in Birmingham constructed by Cadbury's, Port Sunlight in Liverpool by Lever Brothers, Saltaire in Bradford and New Earswick, the construction of Rowntree, were a mixture of paternalism, enlightened reform and an attempt to create an organic village among industrial workers. They were set in rural areas in close proximity to the industrial centre and very often were enclosed communities. They were a part of the Garden City movement that proffered a new idea of combining rural and city life.

Many architects who were later to become famous for their design of expensive middle-class housing worked on these projects mainly out of conviction that a new type of working-class environment could be created (Burnett 1986). Rents were set at a reasonable level, but foremost was the belief that a disciplined and respectable workforce could be created by providing a pleasant and amenable environment. It is not coincidental that most of these schemes were the creation of Quaker families and inherent in them was the humanitarian conviction that people were a product of their environment and that they could be 'saved' from degeneracy and crime. The design of the houses ensured that they were light and airy and were in sharp contrast to the dark and insanitary 'back to back' terraced housing of the cities. Contemporary descriptions sum up the way in which this construction of a model community was viewed:

> (Mr. Cadbury) has built the model village of Bourneville, provided swimming ponds for male and female employees, recreation grounds, cricket and football fields, lawns and shrubberies, gymnasia and reading rooms, besides educational facilities of the most varied description. Indeed, the happiness and health of the workers have ever been the first consideration of the firm. (*Yorkshire Herald* 1906, quoted in Smith 1989:237)

These schemes were essentially different from the towns and communities that had been created around specific industries and occupations. The mining villages and other one-industry areas usually contained a mixture of privately rented and company housing of varying quality. The development of the railways meant that 'railway towns' such as Swindon, Crewe and Darlington were constructed with different types of housing for the various grades of employees. The process of industrialisation meant that working-class people congregated primarily around the sources of work and housing provided mainly by private landlords tended to follow. This was the pattern until the entry of the state into housing provision.

There were many problems involved in the provision of quality housing to the working class, the most pressing was the one of cost. In London especially, rents were high because of the lack of land and the insatiable demand (Burnett 1986). Wages remained static and rent represented a high proportion of the weekly outgoing for the families of the poor.

> Rent increases in a poor area sometimes absorbed the whole of an increase in wages...what is gained in the cost of food goes mainly in additional house rent. (Burnett 1986:151)

Rent was a constant worry in the lives of the poor. As a result of the high cost of renting many people sub-let rooms in houses to other families, which of course further exacerbated overcrowding (Pember Reeves 1913). The problem was further amplified by the necessity for many people to live in the centre of towns where employment was available. Casual work for men and cleaning jobs for women necessitated being close at hand for a start in the early hours of the morning. The poor were immobile, they could not be placed outside where land was relatively cheap, also food prices were lower in central markets and, as Burnett (1986:151) points out, 'debts to local shopkeepers tended to tie the poor to areas where they were known and could obtain credit'. Poverty could be managed on a day-to-day basis as long as the poor remained close to casual work in an area where they had a network of support upon which they could rely in a crisis.

When looking at housing provision prior to state intervention, the divisions within the working classes can be seen to be crucial to an understanding of the problems that were to be faced by local authorities in the future. The cost of housing to both the provider and recipient was the overriding problem. The possession of a secure wage by the 'head of the household', the male breadwinner, was to be the single most important criteria of housing allocation. This in itself served to exclude the very poor, women and the sick and disabled. The immobility of the poor was also a problem as long as casual work existed in the centre of towns. Industrial development had been geographically uneven, which meant that the demand for housing had followed industry and had often led to the rapid growth of low quality house building by speculators.

As Burnett writes, by the end of the nineteenth century, Britain had become a country of town dwellers. Between 1851 and 1911, the total population doubled and the urban population had trebled (Burnett 1978:141). By 1911, nearly 16 million people or about 43 per cent of the population lived in cities with more than 100,000 population. This growth meant that the inadequate provision of housing by private landlords and philanthropic organisations was not sufficient. The state had to intervene to provide.

Ascribing communities before the welfare state

By the 1880s, the housing conditions in large cities, especially London, became the focus of public and political attention. Ironically, the Jack the Ripper murders had focused press attention on to the existence of the foul and dark streets and slums of the East End, known as 'rookeries', within which many of the very poor existed. The popular novels of Charles Dickens also brought home to a middle-class readership the appalling living conditions within towns. Early photographers such as John Thompson published studies of the destitute which are classics today and which attracted much attention at the time.

The East End was the primary focus for concern for social investigators such as Booth, radical socialists such as the Marxists of the Social Democratic Federation and probably, because of its close proximity to the Houses of Parliament, the political establishment. The conditions of the slums were, of course, linked to concerns over public health and public safety and were seen as the site for the growth of moral degeneracy and crime.

State intervention was initially slow throughout the latter part of the century, however, in 1880, the passing of the By-Laws Act marked the first significant move by the state to regulate the design of housing for the masses (see Table 3.1). Housing policies tend to follow two directions, those aimed at the regulations of standards and design of houses, and those which promote the state funding and building of houses. After 1880, 'by-law housing' as it came to be known set the basic standard required for affordable working-class

Table 3.1   State construction of communities 1880–2000

1880	By-law housing – abolition of back-to-back housing, laid down regulations of space and size
1883	Cheap Trains Act – enabled the growth of suburbs – commuting into city to work begins
1890	Housing of the Working Classes Act – empowered Local Authorities to acquire land for building of housing in overcrowded urban areas
1900	Housing of the Working Classes Act – extended powers of purchase to provincial Local Authorities
1918	Tudor Walters Report – set high standards for postwar building of working-class housing
1919	Addison Act – mandatory requirement of Local Authorities to survey housing needs in area and to authorise building. Funded by government subsidy and local rates. Council estates constructed
1924	Wheatley Act – requirement on Local Authorities to raise output of house building. Subsidies increased in order to reduce rents
1930	Greenwood Act – aimed at slum clearance. Housing for the very poor unable to afford high quality council housing. Local Authorities begin to build blocks of flats
1930–39	Growth of suburbs built around new industries – Cowley, Dagenham and Luton for car industry
1939	Barlow Report – recommends construction of New Towns and enlargement of existing small towns
1946	New Towns Act – 12 new towns to be built including Stevenage, Crawley and Harlow
1952	Town Development Act – 'overspill' towns enlarged
1961	Parker Morris Report – recognised growth of working-class affluence. Recommended more space for consumer goods and garages in public housing
1960–70	More New Towns commissioned including Telford and Milton Keynes. Extension of large 'high rise' estates to accommodate demand
1967	Rent Act – control of rents for unfurnished accommodation – to combat slum landlordism – 'Rackmanism'
1974	Housing Act – move towards discretionary sale of council housing by Local Authorities. Emphasis on building 'special needs' housing for elderly
1977	Housing (Homeless Persons Act) – Local Authorities required to house homeless people in area. Categories of priority need established – does not include single homeless – priority to dependent children
1980	Housing Act – the 'Right to Buy' – mandatory requirement on Local Authorities to sell to existing tenants at reduced cost
1988	Housing Act – no more building of houses by Local Authorities. Provision of social housing by Housing Associations
1999	Community Safety Orders – eviction of 'nuisance neighbours' from Local Authority housing
2000	Extension of new housing to 'brown field sites' – old industrial sites and to some 'green belt' areas

housing. This legislation was permissive not mandatory, however, it was a move which set the pattern for future state legislation.

In 1883, the Cheap Trains Act meant that it became feasible for many of the securely employed working class to move from the centre of towns to the suburbs. Consequently many of the new 'by-law' houses began to be built in areas a few miles outside city centres.

> Typically, the by-law housing which spread over large areas of working-class suburbs in London and provincial towns in the late nineteenth century consisted of repetitive terraces of four, eight or more houses.... In those of the better class there might be a tiny front garden with palings to separate the house from the pavement, a bay window and a small rear garden. (Burnett 1986:161)

The old back-to-back terraces were now abolished and replaced by this higher quality housing, but it was obviously only accessible to the upper strata of the working class. The differences in design also followed the social divisions and possession of a front room or a garden became a symbol of class identity.

The provision of housing by local authorities followed. In 1890 the Housing of the Working Classes Act enabled local authorities in large conurbations to acquire land for building and this was followed in 1900 by the extension of these powers to local authorities in the provinces. As Burnett relates, there were two main types of housing which local authorities provided, the blocks of flats in central areas and the cottage estates in the suburbs. The London County Council was the most active, building both types and extending the suburban estates to South London and into Essex and the previously rural areas to the West including Ealing, all of these new suburbs were served by the new Underground and the tram system. Liverpool, Birmingham and Manchester also followed this pattern. Cities were expanding and people were becoming more geographically mobile.

This flurry of building prior to the outbreak of war in 1914 however was a part of a political programme. As Swenarton (1981) argues, much of the growth was under Labour or radical Liberal councils who saw housing as a part of a project of municipal socialism, Conservative councils were far more reluctant to build public housing.

The traumatic social upheaval caused by the 1914–18 war, meant that the housing and the health of the working classes became targeted for reform.

> The first point at which the attack must be delivered is the unhealthy, ugly, overcrowded house in the mean street, which all of us know too well. If a healthy race is to be reared, it can be reared only in healthy homes; if drink and crime are to be successfully combatted, decent sanitary houses must be provided; if 'unrest' is to be converted to contentment, the provision of good houses may prove one of the most potent agents in that conversion. (King's speech reported in *The Times*, 1919, quoted in Burnett 1986:219)

It is fairly obvious from the tone of this speech that the fear of class discontent and even revolution was a background against which the famous 'Homes Fit For Heroes' political manifesto was launched in 1919.

In the immediate aftermath of the war, there was a housing shortage caused by the returning servicemen forming new families, the restriction of building during the war years and the increase in demand from workers in war industries. The following years were marked by an extension in the state responsibility for both the standard and the provision of housing for the working classes. In 1918, the Tudor Walters Act set high standards of space and size for council housing. This was followed in 1919 by the Addison Act, which contained a mandatory requirement of local authorities to survey the housing needs of the area and to authorise building. The building of council estates was to be funded by government subsidy and local rates. In 1924, the first minority Labour government extended the amount of state subsidy in order to reduce rents.

By the 1930s, slum clearance schemes were adopted by many local authorities in large urban areas and housing for the very poor now became a priority. Although the early years of the 1930s was marked by economic depression and mass unemployment, it must be remembered that this was geographically uneven. The areas based upon the traditional industries of coal, steel and ship-building were devastated by the depression. In South Wales, the North-East and in Scotland, whole communities existed on the edge of starvation. The depiction of the hopeless misery of these areas in books such as Orwells' *Road to Wigan Pier* (1937), and films like *Love on the Dole* (1938), reached a wide audience. But at the same time, other areas were in the process of development and rapid change. New industries, such as the car industry, based upon mass production methods were appearing in the Midlands and the South of England. These new industries had a great demand for labour and were situated in previously rural areas such as the Morris Cowley works at Oxford, and the giant Ford factory at Dagenham. Vast housing estates were built to accommodate the new workers and this brought into being a new type of 'company town', ascribed communities reliant on one employer. But, as we shall see, the allocation of housing was dependent upon male employment. The expansion of the new light industries also created new trading estates in the suburbs such as Slough in West London, which in turn led to an expansion of council housing. Moving to the suburbs however required a reasonable income, and there was a famous public health report in Stockton in 1934 when the medical officer of health reported deteriorating health standards on the new estates due to the increase in rents (McGonigle and Kirby 1936).

Despite the great expansion of public housing, therefore, the seeds of the traditional problem of affording good quality housing remained a problem for sections of the working class, 'the rents of the new council houses were such that the link between low incomes and poor accommodation was left largely intact' (Cole and Furbey 1994:51). The new council estates were therefore filled largely by the relatively secure and well-paid working-class families, leaving the slum clearance schemes to cope with the poor and poorest. The social divisions within the working classes that had existed since industrialisation remained intact.

As we have seen, the advent of the Second World War with large-scale evacuation from the urban slums to rural areas vividly illustrated the effects of the appalling living conditions to the concerned middle classes. The 'housing problem' once again became an important postwar public and political issue. The effects of the Blitz in 1940 on large cities such as Plymouth, Coventry, and of course, London, meant that significant sections of working-class people were rendered permanently homeless. To social reformers this was the ideal opportunity to 'build again'. The aspiration to conquer the 'giant' of squalor was of course, embedded in the Beveridge Plan (1942), the blueprint for the postwar welfare state.

Ascribed communities, social democracy and the welfare state

It is estimated that three quarters of a million homes were destroyed or severely damaged by the Second World War and families returning from evacuation and men and women from service overseas increasingly faced homelessness. The mood of early post-war Britain was very much at odds with this situation. The promise of a better future and of an end to the prewar poverty and squalor had swept the Labour Party to power in 1945. The building of this 'New Jerusalem' had no place in it for the urban slums or the cramped and unhealthy housing which had existed since industrialisation. The Labour Party, elected in 1945, had a deep commitment to the implementation of the Beveridge Plan that involved the Keynesian philosophy of state investment and control. The responsibility for the building of new houses was therefore to be the primary responsibility of the state. An 'ambitious council building programme was launched with a target of 240,000 units a year' (Power 1993: 186). Local authorities, therefore, who were already the largest group of landlords, became dominant in postwar housing provision.

The existence of the designated green belt around cities meant that any large-scale building programme had to take place within the city limits or at a location far removed. There were two main directions for tackling the housing shortage and constructing a new Britain, one was for massive slum clearance programmes in industrial urban areas, the other was for the building of New Towns in previously non-urban areas. Both of these policies were to transform the domestic landscape of Britain. The Abercrombie Plan for Greater London published in 1944, proposed both of these solutions to the housing problem. Firstly, it argued for the rebuilding of high density housing in inner cities but these were to be in modern tower block flats rather than in terraced back-to-back housing, and the building of New Towns which were deemed to be specifically suitable for young families.

The New Towns Act of 1946 proposed the building of 20 new towns of which 14 were started between 1947 and 1950. The majority of this first wave of New Towns such as Bracknell, Harlow and Stevenage were intended to accommodate people from the Greater London area. The intention from the outset was that of the creation of new communities. The recommendation of the Committee appointed to set up the towns was clear on 'the guiding principles upon which such Towns should be established and developed as self-contained and balanced communities for work and living' (Osborn and Whittick 1969:100).

The New Towns represented not only a means of housing provision but also a large-scale project of social engineering. They were designed for occupation by young families who would in many respects exemplify the new Britain but they were also based upon the Beveridge ideal of the nuclear family. In some ways the first inhabitants of the New Towns were regarded as pioneers and the move from the familiar overcrowded neighbourhoods of London to the relative isolation of the New Towns was the subject of much academic and media attention. The first British television soap opera 'The Grove Family' was set in such a town and chronicled the move of a London family. The move especially affected the lives of women, who with young families often found themselves alienated and lonely. In a study of Harlow, nicknamed 'Pram Town' by the press due to its high birth rate, Attfield chronicles the feeling of the young women,

> I knew a lot of women that moved down here...we all moved together and some of them suffered terribly with depression and loneliness although there was a better sense of community than there is now...the women were the ones that was left to cope and adjust, harder than any of the men. (Attfield 1989:215)

The result of such a feeling created a new public health problem, that of 'New Town blues' with the reported hospitalisation of women with mental neuroses in one New Town, being 50 per cent higher than the national average.

Nevertheless, the building of New Towns continued throughout the 1950s and the 1960s under both Labour and Conservative administrations. A second wave was constructed in the late 1960s including Milton Keynes, Telford, Washington and Cwmbran in Wales, and Livingstone in Scotland. After 1967, the expansion of existing towns was undertaken, this move affected Northampton, Swindon and many others whose population doubled and sometimes trebled within a decade.

New Towns represented the ideal of a constructed 'community'. People were forced to set up new social networks to replace the traditional links of the extended family. Within unfamiliar modernistic and functional settings the lives of many working-class people were transformed. During the 1960s and 1970s, employment was high and the new industries based upon technical, light engineering and white-collar jobs ensured a relatively high standard of living.

The alternative policy of the rebuilding of inner cities and the construction of high rise flats and estates was also to transform working-class lives and culture. But within the plans for new estates and high rise developments, one factor remained stable, the ideal of the male-breadwinner and the nuclear family as the occupiers of the new housing. The postwar housing programme was firmly based upon pro-natalist principles dedicated to the raising of the birth rate, and decent housing was seen as the inducement to women to fulfil their role of motherhood. As Roberts (1991) vividly demonstrates not only was the design of houses based upon the ideal of the full-time home-based wife and mother, the rents of houses were calculated on the average male wage. But within this gendered division of allocation, the postwar Labour government sought to make council housing classless. The idea was for 'mixed development', that meant a diversity of housing, flats for single people and houses for families, but also a social mix. Bevan, the Minister for Housing as well as Health, argued that communities should represent a 'living tapestry' in which all social classes would live in proximity (Roberts 1991:57). But as we shall see, in reality the old divisions within the working class were reinforced by local authority allocation policies.

Most local authorities operated a point system of allocation based upon need, but this was accompanied by an informal system whereby the 'respectable' working class were allocated to the new prestigious flagship estates. Criteria such as standards of housekeeping, a respectable reputation and a good record of tenancy as well as unrecognised racism were all applied by individual housing officers (Power 1987). This was recognised by people themselves and certain estates gained the reputation of being 'superior'. The tenants themselves often perceived of the situation in this way;

See . . . years ago it was a struggle to move onto this estate, they were selective they had a bit of . . . without actually being told there was discrimination

Because, I would say, without being, you know, snooty the tenants were selected. Like getting into a school there is selection isn't there? And we thought it was good, yes, good.

One woman, who was Irish and married to an unskilled labourer and had six children, implicitly recognised the informal racism of selection,

I think I was very lucky to get this place. (Quoted in Roberts 1991:124/5)

The status divisions within the working class were being both reinforced and were in process of change during the 1960s and early 70s (Goldthorpe and Lockwood 1969, Stacey 1970). On the one hand, the good estates offered a 'respectable life' to the traditional working class, but the newly affluent workers were also effecting change. The move to New Towns and new estates by the now relatively highly paid manual workers also meant a change in cultural attitudes. The proliferation of consumer goods such as television, fitted carpets and new furniture meant that 'moving to the front' became common place.

The move to the front was a symbolic gesture which represented a new consumerism (Zweig 1961). The move to the new suburban estates encouraged 'home-centredness' and the 'public' life of the pre-war poor working-class communities was being replaced by a more private emphasis on home life and individual achievement. There was a recognition by policy-makers that working-class aspirations and cultures were significantly changed, for in 1961 the Parker Morris Report (Ministry of Housing 1961) set out high standards for new public and private housing which included more floor space, larger kitchens and garages.

The building of tower blocks of flats was very much a feature of the 1960s. They appeared to be the solution for increased demand for housing following from accelerated slum clearance schemes. Flats, although popular with single people and childless couples, were disliked by families. High-rise flats were often built on estates designated as 'overspill' and did not have the social status of the green estates. But many local authorities, especially in England, continued to build flats and they represented 55 per cent of all tenders approved by 1964 (Burnett 1986:301). The Ronan Point disaster in 1968, which saw the collapse of a tower block in central London, effectively brought to an end their institutional popularity. By 1970, the tower block was effectively abandoned as a form of housing provision.

When looking at this brief postwar picture of the construction of ascribed communities, one salient factor stands out, the connection between housing development, communities, and full employment. The new communities constructed by social policies were based upon full male employment, the home-based housewife (who by the late 1960s was increasingly employed part time), the nuclear family and economic stability and security. Many of the older estates that had been in existence since the 1930s were also based around one industry and even one employer. As a recent article about the Ford's Becontree Estate in Essex recalls;

> Over the last 65 years every member of my family has worked there . . . . the factory's fortunes and three-shift system imposed the rhythm of life on everyone I grew up with. (Lashmar 2000)

The New Towns and the new council estates built during the 1950s and 1960s were to a lesser extent based upon one industry but were based upon the ideal of the male breadwinner even though many of the new light industries which employed a female workforce were set up in proximity to them. The social divisions within the working class were also reinforced by allocation policies and increased affluence meant a change in traditional cultures. The postwar welfare state was the background to the construction of ascribed communities. As Chen noted, citizenship had been constructed as a belonging to this new social democracy based upon equality of opportunity and full employment. Although gender divisions remained deeply entrenched and immigration was beginning to reinforce and construct forms of institutionalised racism, nevertheless, one can see this period between 1945 and 1975, as the high point of welfarism. But, by the mid 1970s, economic security was faltering and full employment was becoming a thing of the past.

Consumerism, social polarisation and ascribed communities

During the 1980s and 1990s many of the taken-for-granted assumptions about the competency and desirability of the welfare state to provide protection from 'cradle to grave' were shattered. Many people who had grown up with the certainties of the welfare state were catapulted into a challenging and, at times, threatening environment. But this period also brought new-found wealth and affluence to many others. The decades between 1980 and the close of the century saw British society fragment and polarise.

This period was politically dominated by a New Right agenda that believed passionately in the power of the market and rejected the role of the state as the provider of welfare and security. The identity of 'citizen' of the welfare state that had been constructed in the postwar years was replaced by that of 'consumer' within a market system. This redefinition, as we have seen in Chapter 2, was also taking place in health policies at the this time.

This new direction in housing policies revolutionised the position and social composition of public housing. Housing policies, with their emphasis on ownership rather than tenancy, both reinforced existing social divisions and spatially constructed polarised communities which increasingly became sites of social exclusion. The one policy that had the greatest impact on the process of residualisation of council housing and the polarisation of communities was the 1980 'Right to Buy' legislation.

As many writers (Forrest and Murie 1988) have noted, the first Thatcher administration did not initiate the sale of council housing, this had been an ongoing process since 1960. Sales had however remained low during the 1960s, but in 1972 the Conservative government had encouraged purchasing and had also presided over the decline in the building of new houses. In 1972, sales of council houses reached a record 45,878 (Forrest and Murie 1988:110). But these sales were at the discretion of local authorities, the 'Right to Buy' legislation made the sale of council housing compulsory. This was to have the twin effect of residualisation and marginalisation. As well as selling council housing stock, no new housing was to be built by local authorities. This meant that existing council housing was either sold or became a residual provision for the socially marginalised. Between 1980 and 1984, over half a million houses were sold to sitting tenants (Forrest and Murie 1988:110). Sales were not uniform throughout the country, there were high rates of sales in the South East of England, the East Midlands and the South West but London had a relatively low take-up. In Scotland, Glasgow had the lowest sales and in Wales, sales were concentrated in the more affluent areas of Cardiff, Swansea and Newport. There were many factors influencing sales, proximity to privately owned estates, area, the quality of housing, for instance. Houses which had been built to high standards in the 1950s were very popular but high-rise flats were not.

The sale of council housing illustrated existing social divisions within the working class. Areas that had been highly sought after and had had strict allocation policies, the desirable green estates which housed the settled, affluent and respectable working class, were the ones most likely to be purchased. The high rise blocks and out of town estates which had been the centre of slum clearance schemes were the least likely to be purchased. The 'typical' purchaser was,

> a long established tenant, in middle age, with a fairly large family grown up, earning above average wages, in a skilled manual occupation and often with more than one wage earner in the household. (Forrest and Murie 1988:172)

Research showed that this model was consistent throughout Britain. It is noticeable that the pattern of basing allocation on the nuclear family with a male breadwinner in the 1950s and 60s was to be reflected in the purchasing of the 1980s. It is also important to note that this model excludes many other groups and so the pre-existing social divisions were concretised by the purchasing of council houses. The respectable working-class family which had been the model for the Beveridgean welfare state, became consumers and home owners, but this meant that others were to be left outside and this marginalisation was to be spatial as well as social. Sections of the working class began to move away from the council estates, and resales of purchased houses went to young first-time buyers, mostly families with small children. The best of the council housing stock had been sold by the end of the 1980s, leaving local authorities with the worst houses or flats on the least attractive estates with which to meet the needs of the most socially and economically deprived people. These estates became characterised by the population left behind,

> In terms of social composition, those remaining in council housing are generally very poor, young with young children, unemployed, elderly retired or single person households. (Flynn 1988:300)

Not only are the poor and relatively deprived social groups now confined to council housing, the houses and the estates themselves have deteriorated, sometimes to the point of dereliction. Throughout the 1980s, local authorities could not spend revenue on repairs to council housing and, by 1986, an Audit Commission report calculated that the cost of outstanding repairs would be over £10 million. Flynn accurately describes a typical estate that has become a familiar sight in most of Britain,

> Many of the worst housing estates are reserved by the local authority for 'problem cases' which marks both the tenants and the estate out in the wider locality. These estates deteriorate still further due to poor social amenities: chemists move out

because of break-ins; new health clinics can rarely find suitable space; shops and cheaper supermarkets, along with leisure and sports centres, are rarely built on council estates...and the police are more likely to treat residents as potential criminals rather than as potential victims. (Flynn, quoted in Mann 1992:101)

In many aspects this description is reminiscent of those of the slums and warrens vividly illustrated by Victorian observers. These are Britain's 'dangerous places' that have become the province of a designated 'underclass' of the socially excluded. Those who have no social or economic power; the poor, long-term unemployed, chronically sick or disabled, people released from long-term care, single mothers and children, state pensioners, are often allocated to these 'hard to let' estates. They too comprise an ascribed community of a specific type.

Local authorities, as we have seen, were the predominant providers and landlords of social housing from the interwar years until the 1980s. But this role was to be changed by housing legislation designed to lessen the power and responsibilities of local government and to change its function from that of provider to enabler. This change in role was a part of the universal move towards a mixed economy in welfare epitomised by the NHS and Community Care Act of 1990. The sector which was given the responsibility for providing 'social' housing was the housing associations. The 1988 Housing Act stressed the enabling role of local government and the increased importance of housing associations that were seen as belonging in the 'private' sector, as the main providers of housing for those unable to afford to buy on the market. The roots of housing associations lie in the charitable and voluntary organisations of the nineteenth century and as Lund (1996) argues, their identity was transformed following the 1988 Housing Act. Tenants of housing association properties were regarded as those of private landlords and the rents charged were required to meet market levels. Therefore the tenants, who by definition were poor, needed housing benefit in order to afford the rents. A further step towards the removal of local government from the management of social housing came in 1989 under the Local Government and Housing Act. Under this Act, local authorities could undertake the 'voluntary transfer' of their existing housing stock to other agencies including private landlords and housing associations and tenants were given the right to opt for alternative landlords. The remaining responsibility of local authorities was to house the homeless. Under agreements with housing associations, however, local authorities retained a percentage of the allocation of tenancies and therefore housing association developments included a section for those who were regarded as priority for rehousing.

Housing Associations throughout Britain are multi-financed, they receive grants from local authorities, investment from the market and revenue from rents. They build new houses on estates, or in specific roads on existing private estates, in isolated rows in rural and urban areas, or they take over the management of existing properties where the owners are experiencing financial

difficulties. The social impact of the housing legislation of the late 1980s has
been to further polarise localities. The requirement on housing associations to
move away from their traditional role in the provision of 'special needs' housing to family housing which must be provided at a market rent
has meant that 'many associations are building new estates of family housing
with rents at such levels that they are not affordable to those working and in
receipt of low incomes' (Harriott and Matthews 1998:246). Thus, many of
the new estates or strips of houses resemble 'benefit' ghettoes consisting of
those who are not in the labour market; single mothers, long-term unemployed, chronic sick and disabled and pensioners. The houses therefore may
be new but the social composition of the tenants remains that of the socially
deprived.

At the same time as the emergence of 'sink' estates and benefit ghettoes,
there was an increase in owner-occupation and the proliferation of private
housing estates throughout Britain. By the end of 1998, over 2.3 million
council houses and New Town Development Corporation houses had been
transferred to individual ownership. Altogether, in the years between 1961 and
1998, the number of owner-occupied dwellings had doubled (to 16.9 million)
and correspondingly the number of rented dwellings had fallen by a sixth
(Social Trends 2000:168). By the end of the twentieth century, Britain had
the highest rate of owner-occupation (68 per cent) in the European Union
(Social Trends 30 2000:168). This growth in consumerism in housing also
had the effect of widening the social composition of ownership in one aspect
at least, that of family type. By 1998, the numbers of couples taking out new
mortgages on houses had fallen from 74 per cent in 1983 to 58 per cent, and,
correspondingly, the numbers of single-women new mortgagees had risen dramatically from 8 per cent in 1983 to 18 per cent in 1998. The singles market
now represents nearly 50 per cent of new housing and housing developments
in all areas reflect this social change. These developments are now targeted
at specific groups such as 'starter homes' for first-time buyers, retirement
villages for wealthy over-50s, city apartments and lofts for young single
urban professionals, and 'executive' detached houses for growing families.
Within many large cities, old docklands were scheduled for redevelopment
and were transformed from previously derelict and poverty-stricken areas
into smart and expensive housing and leisure facilities, this is a feature of
all old working docks in London, Liverpool, Cardiff, Bristol and many
other places. All of these new typologies of housing are marketed to appeal
to a consumerist identity. People are now defined and define themselves
as belonging to diversified consumer groups rather than as members of a
social strata defined by class. This is, sociologically, a new factor in the definition of groups within the population. These could be described as *elective*
communities, with people actively choosing (and possessing the social power
to choose) to identify with certain group traits and characteristics. But there
are other communities which exhibit elements of both ascribed and elective
definitions.

Ascribed, elective and marginalised communities

We now turn to look briefly at three very different types of 'community' which exhibit aspects of being both ascribed and elective and which, in varying ways, illustrate the difficulty of understanding the term 'community'. This chapter began by looking at the many ways in which the phrase 'community' is used to denote both a locality and a social and cultural identity and how the two are frequently entangled. If we take the three examples of: minority ethnic groups, rural inhabitants, and the homeless, the inter-connection of cultural diversity, social power and inequality within social policies can be seen to operate to create the identity of a 'community'. The minority ethnic and the rural communities were in some way *ascribed* to specific areas within a historical juncture but may now be said to *elect* to identify culturally and socially with the locality. The advent of visible homelessness on the streets of large cities during the 1980s caused public and political concern but was this situation a response to policies and social and economic upheaval which was beyond the control of individuals?

The presence of minority ethnic communities in Britain has a long history. The first group of identifiable size was probably the Irish who could be said to have literally built the canals, railways and factories of Britain during the Industrial Revolution. As Mann reports, the majority were unskilled peasants who 'left abject rural poverty in Ireland for the relatively rich cities of Northern Britain' (Mann 1992:37). The Irish, as we saw in Chapter 1, were the subject of discrimination and segregation and suspected of being carriers of infectious diseases. They were the poorest section of the working class and lived in the worst conditions in the worst slums of the large cities such as Liverpool where they settled for work. They were the subject of anti-Catholic hatred and often violence that exists, to some extent, to the present day. The political situation in Northern Ireland and the resultant bombings in mainland Britain further exacerbated the anti-Irish culture in Britain during the 1960s and 1970s. The social and economic position of the Irish population in Britain remains fairly low. They continue to be over-represented in unskilled manual work and to have relatively low health status (McKeigue 1991). There are still definable Irish communities in most large cities, their area of 'settlement' was determined by proximity to work and its cultural identification has been constructed over time. Likewise, many urban areas have identifiable Jewish communities which also have a long history of settlement in areas that offered a place of work and opportunities to expand. Like the Catholic Irish, Jewish communities are defined by locality and strong cultural identity.

The postwar welfare state increased the demand for labour, and immigration from former colonies and empire also increased to meet demand. This immigration came mainly from two sources, the West Indies and the Indian subcontinent. Britain, unlike the rest of Europe, never coordinated housing and immigration policy. As the welfare state was expanding to offer a measure of security in the council housing sector to the respectable 'white' working class, so the 'non-white' population was effectively excluded:

many local authorities (on a variety of pretexts but most notably via residence requirements) refused to house black people. Even by the mid 1960s, only 6% of the overseas-born black population as compared with 28% Irish migrants and a third of the English-born had been accommodated in this sector, despite black peoples' lower than average incomes and greater apparent need. (Rose et al. 1969, quoted in Smith 1989:52)

This exclusion from public sector housing for those on the lowest incomes and often victims of racial discrimination, left the migrants with two alternatives; private renting or house purchase. By the 1960s, private renting was the predominant form of tenure of Afro-Caribbean households and, as Rex and Moore (1967) described in their famous study, this was confined to older dilapidated housing in inner cities, which they called 'twilight zones'. House purchase was an increasing option for many, but the houses purchased were old and in the least desirable streets of inner cities. Although on low incomes, mortgages were often obtained via private moneylenders at high rates, and they were doubly penalised as they did not receive tax concessions. Nevertheless, by the end of the 1960s, 33 per cent of black Londoners and 60 per cent of those in the West Midlands were home-owners, while only 4 per cent and 6 per cent had secured a council tenancy (Rose et al. 1969). Like all new migrants, many chose to move to areas where they had friends and relations and where work was readily available. This explains the concentration of minority ethnic communities in Britain today, with London and the West Midlands being the two conurbations with the highest concentration of communities. But there are wide variations in these areas, with most Afro-Caribbeans concentrated in outer London areas and the Pakistani and Bangladeshi communities more concentrated in the West Midlands. The Indian and Chinese communities are much more dispersed. Recent research (Policy Studies Institute 1998) has shown that although 'white' people tend to live in areas of low ethnic minority population, even in deprived areas, other groups, notably Pakistani and Bangladeshi people, live in areas of high concentration of minority ethnic groups. They are also most likely to live in deprived wards in all areas. Owner-occupation increases concentration of population as streets and areas become predominantly owned by one group but this conversely can also be a sign of greater deprivation and poverty. The housing required by the larger extended families within these communities can only be obtained through overcrowding or the buying of small terraced houses in a row. Unlike 'white' population, home-ownership for the majority of the 'black' population is associated with poverty, bad housing and social deprivation. There is one exception to this picture, that of an increasing number of South Asians in London who are building 'communities of relative affluence' (Policy Studies Institute 1998). On the whole, however, the majority of people of the minority ethnic communities, but especially those for whom the Muslim religion is an important identifier, live in relative deprivation. The reasons are multi-complex but inner city location is one that tends to be a general factor. The association of urban and especially inner city areas with high deprivation, crime levels and poverty is one of the causal factors in the 'white flight' to the suburbs and rural areas.

The romantic appeal of the village has dominated English culture and been a significant factor in housing design this century. Within the English culture, the country has connotations of purity and innocence but the town or city is associated with danger and dirt (Williams 1975). The 'village in the mind' was a causal factor in the increase in the so-called 'gentrification' of the countryside that became a demographic trend in the 1960s (Pahl 1965). A section of the urban middle-classes began to move out of towns and to buy properties in rural areas that were close enough to make commuting possible. The construction of the 'dormitory suburb' and the 'commuter village' was the result of such moves. These areas, as their name suggests, were not a village 'community' in the traditional sense but enclaves of middle-class families who were only in residence in the evenings and at weekends. The social significance of this phenomenon was great, property prices rose dramatically. In the absence of much public housing for rent many of the original inhabitants could no longer afford to remain. The social and economic class divisions between the incomers and the 'real villagers' were immense (Newby 1985). This situation was repeated throughout many areas, the most notable being in Essex and East Anglia in England and in North Wales. In Wales, the situation was further compounded by the fact that most of the 'incomers' were English and the marginalised locals were Welsh. The buying of second homes in country areas by wealthy urbanites further exacerbated local housing shortages and in some instances caused tension and even violent protest. Within many rural areas today, a distinct pattern can be seen with the construction of two distinct 'communities', the relatively wealthy professional people, sometimes retired, who have bought and renovated property in the area and the indigent population, who strive to work in a declining agricultural sector.

By the late 1990s, Britain was suffering an agricultural depression. Due to the BSE (commonly called 'mad cow disease') crisis and increased competition, farm prices for meat reached an all time low. The romantic view of country living began to fade, with suicide rates highest among the farming 'community'. The extent of rural poverty is difficult to quantify as total numbers in the population are much smaller than in urban areas. A recent study of rural poverty noted that; low pay is more prevalent in rural areas, unemployment rates are similar to urban areas but there is a high number (23 per cent) who are self-employed on low incomes and exempt from some benefits, and 41 per cent are not in the labour market at all (Joseph Rowntree Foundation 1998). In addition to this, many of those who are employed live in 'tied' housing. The privately rented sector is much larger in rural areas with one in seven households living in rented accommodation – 50 per cent more than in urban areas (JRF 1995). Many rural communities are therefore a mixture of affluence and hidden isolated poverty. These divisions are as deep as in urban areas and the idea of the village as a 'tapestry' containing a diversity of social classes is in many ways a myth. But one phenomenon exclusive to towns and cities which was created during the 1980s was the spectacle of homeless people sleeping rough on the streets and begging publicly.

Homelessness was of course not a 'new' problem, there had been descriptions of the homeless on the streets in Victorian literature and the squatter campaigns that followed both world wars had focused upon the issue. But with the advent of the postwar welfare state and universalist housing policies, the problem had been sidelined as primarily a welfare one. This changed in the mid 1960s, when the television play *Cathy Come Home* was shown in 1966, causing a public outcry. The play depicted the plight of an ordinary working-class family made homeless by a combination of inadequate housing provision and bad luck. The ensuing political concern led to the setting up of the housing charity and pressure group, Shelter, to campaign on behalf of the homeless. At the time, the official figure of homeless families living in temporary accommodation was approximately 2500 households, but by the beginning of the 1990s, it was estimated that homelessness was affecting approximately half a million people (Skellington 1993). What had caused this extraordinary increase? And who are the homeless?

Homelessness historically had not been perceived primarily as a housing issue but as a social welfare one. Throughout the 1950s and 1960s, homeless people were not likely to be housed by local authorities as the prime target of housing departments was people living in slum conditions rather than people who were actually homeless. The link between homelessness and alcoholism, mental illness, prostitution and other social problems was often made by housing departments reluctant to take responsibility for those who were not considered 'deserving' or 'suitable' for council accommodation. Children of the homeless would be taken in to care (this was the plot of *Cathy Come Home*) but the responsibility of local authorities did not extend to adults. This changed with the 1977 Housing (Homeless Persons) Act.

This Act, for the first time, created categories of the homeless and set out priority criteria for rehousing by local authorities. As Skellington (1993) records, this Act contained all the negative views and ideologies concerning the identity and 'deserving' nature of the homeless. Historically, the role of local authorities had been to provide housing for working-class families who could not afford to buy or were renting privately and living in substandard accommodation. But this changed with the Act and now they were being required to house those who had never before presented a claim on housing departments. One officer summed up the feelings of many, 'I have to pay attention to the ordinary standards of decent people. We don't want these dead-legs. They muck up the books and make life a misery for ordinary folk' (Thompson 1988:2).

But through the wording of the Act, the official definition of homelessness was constructed and brought into being a definable category of the population. Homelessness was defined as the 'lack of secure accommodation, free from violence or the threat of violence'. The homeless then fell into four main categories: homeless as defined in the Act; a priority group which was families with children and pregnant women; emergency cases (young people leaving care, ex-psychiatric patients) or people 'at risk' either because of old age or disability. A further two important categories were also applied, a person must not be seen to have made themselves 'intentionally homeless' (this was often applied to women fleeing domestic violence) and must have a local connection with the area. This legislation defined homelessness as lacking 'accommodation' rather than a home which meant that families living in squalid bed and breakfast hostels were not always judged to be 'in need'.

During the late 1970s and early 1980s, unemployment soared and many people who previously would have been able to afford private rented accommodation could no longer afford to do so. Applications for council housing grew at precisely the same time as the 'Right to Buy' policy was introduced – the best of the existing stock was sold and there was very little new building. In addition, policies preceding the community care legislation of 1990 saw the closure of large long-stay mental institutions and childrens' homes which increased the number of vulnerable and desperate people seeking housing. This caused a crisis in street homelessness, with an ever-increasing number of people with nowhere to go. As Power (1993) reports, the demands on depleted council housing stock was unprecedented and the social composition of housing estates began to change. By 1990, nearly half of all Afro-Caribbean households were in council accommodation, mostly flats on 'hard to let' estates. The situation deteriorated throughout the 1980s, as the 1977 Act began to take effect,

> Access for the most needy was guaranteed by legislation, as long as people fitted the legal definition. Councils had little choice but to go 'down market'. Those that were excluded, such as young, single people often resorted to the streets. (Power 1993:231)

As we can see, therefore, the category of 'homeless' became complex and multi-layered, with a hierarchy developing between those who managed to gain low-quality council housing on 'hard to let' estates characterised by high rates of crime and deprivation and those who, failing to gain even this toehold, went on the streets.

There were three further factors which helped to increase the numbers of young single people who emerged onto the streets in most towns and cities after the mid 1980s: the increase in youth unemployment; the break up of many families which often left teenagers in homes with abusive relationships and the erosion of all state benefits, but especially those to 16 to 18 year olds which left many literally with no income. The result of many such factors was the public spectacle of street begging and sleeping rough in doorways that were familiar urban sights by the 1990s. As well as the young, the mentally ill, drug users and men discharged from the services following cutbacks in the Armed forces all found their way to areas which became locally well known and took on the appearance of medieval encampments. As Sir George Young, the then Housing Minister, famously remarked in 1991, 'Homeless people are the sort you tread on when you come out of the opera' (quoted in *The Mail on Sunday* 1991).

One mental health charity, Concern, estimated that 40 per cent of homeless people were suffering from a form of mental illness, and this began to be a cause of publicised concern over the 'mad on the streets', The description of 'the homeless' began to be applied to all categories of street dwellers, and they became increasingly stigmatised as an alien community,

Not only are those who happen to have nowhere to live being attributed a 'nature' (poor, financially incapable, black, beaten up, undeserving) they are now a 'population', citizens presumably of another country. (Roof 1990)

But homeless people did not really form a 'community', they were fragmented and, although it tended to be mentally ill people who gained the publicity, it was the presence of young 'runaways' on the streets that caused equally greater concern. In 1996, concern over this group deepened when housing benefit to those under the age of 25 was further reduced and the duty of local authorities to provide permanent housing for the 'statutory homeless' was to be removed. At Centrepoint in Central London, a large hostel catering for young people between 16 and 25, it was reported that, 'Nearly four out of ten people . . . were 17 years or younger and 48 per cent were either black or from ethnic minorities' (*The Independent* 1996:7).

The charity further reported in the same survey, that the main reasons why young people left home were abuse and family breakdown. Young people from minority ethnic groups are over-represented among the young single homeless. A survey in 1996 found that 26 per cent of all residents in hostels or bed and breakfast accommodation are from minority ethnic groups and that 44 per cent of 16 and 17 year olds and 28 per cent of the under 25s are black (Strong 1996:18). Strong describes this as the 'hidden homeless', young people especially from Asian communities who do not sleep rough on the streets (because of vulnerability to racial attack) but who nevertheless remain homeless within their own communities. There have been a number of initiatives to address the problem of the young single homeless including the foyer schemes which operate in many areas under the auspices of housing associations and in 1998 'rough sleeping' became one of the problems to be addressed by the Social Exclusion Unit.

We have looked briefly at three different types of 'communities' that could be said to be both ascribed and elective. We began this chapter by looking at the way in which working-class and, to a lesser extent, middle-class communities were ascribed by social policies before and throughout the welfare state. The pre and postwar council estates were filled with working-class families who fulfilled the Beveridge ideal of the male breadwinner and female carer model upon which the welfare state was founded. But the underpinning of this model of social democracy was full male employment and a secure industrial

Figure 3.3 Divisions and cultural identities

Ascribed	*Elective*	*Marginalised*
Class-based Production	Income-based Consumption	Existence
Homogeneous	Heterogeneous	Homogeneous
Role specific	Role diverse	Role specific
Geographically-centered locality	Cultural	Locality of shared need
Externally constructed	Voluntaristic	Externally-constructed Individual response
Occupation based	Lifestyle	Uniformity of situation
Civic/individualised culture	Civic/group culture	Individualised/deviant culture
Traditional working class Middle-class suburbs	Gay community Student community	Homeless Drug-users

economy. As great economic, cultural and social change swept through Britain after the 1970s and in a more uncertain context, fears about the 'decline' of community gained publicity. The increase in consumerism, regional economic decline, unemployment, divorce and single-parent families and multiculturalism, have all had an effect on the taken-for-granted assumptions of the old model of social citizenship in stable ascribed communities.

The typology of communities (Figure 3.1) with which this chapter began now requires amendment and finer tuning to illustrate the multi-dimensional and intra-group and locality divisions which have been constructed in the last 20 years (see Figure 3.3).

By the late 1990s, the social problems experienced by many in dangerous estates and on the streets, the poverty of children, lack of opportunities for young people and the plight of the elderly were being addressed by a New Labour government who placed the notion of 'community' at the centre of social policies to eradicate social exclusion.

Social exclusion, communitarianism and policies

We began this chapter by arguing that community is both a locality and a means of cultural identification. The construction of ascribed and elective communities through cumulative social policies allowed people to identify their belonging to a 'community' with a locality and a way of life. But there were always those who remained excluded and marginalised. Until recently,

the phrase social exclusion was virtually unknown outside of political and academic circles. The term of the 'underclass' was one with which most people
would have been familiar. The underclass debate was initially formed in the
USA and is primarily associated with the writer Charles Murray. In the context of the USA, Murray posited a view of a segment of society (mainly urban
blacks) who were completely segregated from the mainstream of society and
did not share the values, traditions or beliefs of the respectable working classes.
(Murray 1990). The blame for the creation of this underclass he placed firmly
on the development of feminism and the welfare system which allowed women
to have children without marriage to a male breadwinner, gave benefits to the
work shy and was too understanding of juvenile offenders. Throughout the
1980s and 90s in Britain, these views gained currency and there were British
sociologists who echoed this analysis of the breakdown of society (Dennis and
Erdos 1993). The current discourse of social exclusion has, therefore, roots in
the effects of the mass unemployment and social and economic change which
many previously secure working-class communities experienced during this
time. In 1997, the incoming New Labour government set up the Social
Exclusion Unit (SEU) which was within the Cabinet and reported directly
to the Prime Minister. However, the concept of 'social exclusion' remains
a contested notion. The definition with which the SEU works is one which
broadens the meaning from just one of 'poverty' to:

> a short-hand label for what can happen when individuals or areas suffer from a con-
> centration of linked problems such as unemployment, poor skills, low income, poor
> housing, high crime, bad health and family breakdown. (SEU 1997)

Others widen the definition still further:

> we are speaking of people who are suffering such a degree of multi-dimensional
> disadvantage, of such duration and reinforced by such material and cultural degra-
> dation of the neighbourhoods in which they live, that their relational links with the
> wider society are ruptured to a degree which is in some considerable degree
> irreversible. (Room 1999)

This recognition of the reality of social exclusion and the need to address its
origins became the underlying objective of government policies on community regeneration that place community nurses in the forefront in partnership
with social workers and voluntary groups. We look in more detail at these policies in Chapter 6. Within all these policies lies the discourse and the central
principle of communitarianism (see Table 3.2).

The concept of communitarianism, like that of the underclass, emerged
from the USA in the 1990s. The ideal of communitarianism was posed by the
American sociologist Etzioni (1995) as the cultural response to the construction of an underclass who were increasingly alienated from mainstream society. But Etzioni saw this alienation as one that was a wider phenomenon than

Table 3.2   Social exclusion, health, community and family 1997–2001

1997	Social Exclusion Unit set up in Cabinet Office, reports directly to Prime Minister
1998	Welfare to Work programme – aimed at 16–25 year olds but includes single mothers of school-age children who are encouraged to return to work
1998	Supporting Families – recommends family-friendly employment policies, SureStart programmes of early intervention to prevent social exclusion, enhanced role for health visitors
1998	The New NHS (England), Putting Patients First (Wales) Designed to Care (Scotland) – End of GP fundholding, replaced by locality commissioning by Primary Care Groups (England), Local Health Groups (Wales)
1998	Appointment of Minister for Public Health, Publication of *Our Healthier Nation* (England), *Better Health-Better Wales* (Wales), *Working Together for a Healthier Scotland* (Scotland). Expansion of public health projects such as Health Action Zones. Recognition of poverty as main cause of ill health
1998	Modernising Social Services – plans for more cooperation between health and social services
1998	National Childcare Strategy – recommends good quality childcare for all under age of 14. Local projects funded, childcare allowances for working single mothers
1999	Modernising Mental Health Services – improvement of services and protection of public, 'community care has failed'
1999	Independent Inquiry into Inequalities in Health (Acheson Report), – poverty single largest cause of ill health – recommends increase in benefits.
1999	Working Families Tax Credit replaces Family Credit. Guaranteed weekly income to those in work
1999	Community Safety Orders – eviction of 'nuisance neighbours' from public housing, curfews on younger children
1999	*With Respect for Old Age* – report by Royal Commission on long-term care. recommends universal free nursing and social care. But minority report recommends means testing for charging for personal care in institutions
1999	Teenage Pregnancy Report by Social Exclusion Unit – increased sex education beginning in primary schools, enhanced role for school nurses, school-aged mothers to continue education
2000	NHS Plan (England) increased funding of NHS but restrictions on private work done by consultants, hospitals judged on efficiency, recruitment of doctors and nurses. Personal care to elderly in residential homes to be charged

just one possessed by the marginalised. Communitarianism argues for a change of emphasis in policies from a concentration upon *rights* to a focus upon *responsibilities and duties*. It is placed in opposition to both the New Right emphasis upon individualism and also to the state welfarism of traditional Labour. By rejecting both previous political philosophies, the emphasis on responsibilities as a part of citizenship has become a part of the 'third way' in social policies of the New Labour government (see Chapter 2). Within this view, communities themselves are seen as the main units of both social organisation and as providers of social care and architects of social cohesion. Policies such as the implementation of Community Safety Orders which allow local authorities and housing associations to evict 'nuisance' neighbours, curfews on younger children and the new category of 'racial harassment' which can be a cause for prosecution and eviction, all point to a determination to enforce responsibilities to the wider community.

Communities are to become the basis of social life, families are strengthened within the overall context of strong and supportive communities. There is an emphasis on self-reliance and self-help but not as an individual characteristic. Instead, groups within communities are encouraged to take responsibility for the provision of services. The role of the voluntary sector, of self-help groups and support networks are enhanced.

> New Labour sell community as the hangover cure to the excesses of Conservative individualism. Community will create social cohesion out of the market culture of self interest. . . . Community will restore the moral balance to society by setting out duties and obligations as well as rights. (Driver and Martell 1997:27)

The role of the professions such as health visitors then becomes one of facilitating rather than delivering services, this is why some writers (Johnson 1999) have argued that communitarianism is essentially anti-professional (we will return to this debate in the next chapter).

Within this emphasis on communities is a high status placed upon the role of the family. Although government spokespeople have been careful to avoid defining a model of 'the family', nevertheless, the consultative document *Supporting Families* (Home Office 1998), stated that 'marriage was the best basis for rearing children and that 'the family was at the heart of our society'. However, this rhetoric is not simply a return to 'basics', it does contain a new view of society and of the roles of men and women. Underlying policies is the commitment to the value of work as the route to social inclusion and citizenship. For the first time, this is applied to women as well as men and to mothers of school-aged children. So what are the responsibilities of citizens in the new welfare state? Basically they are to work, to be involved in civic life in the community and to raise responsible families within which children reach their potential through education and future employment. But this ideal requires the construction of social cohesion in communities and localities that are, at present, socially excluded. It is this construction of social cohesion that will involve branches of community nursing. The policy objectives of active citizenship and social inclusion demand an overall vision and 'joined-up' working. This will mean a change of role and identity for community nurses and it is these changes that are the focus of discussion in Chapter 4 and Chapter 5.

Summary

This chapter has attempted to illustrate the construction of communities in terms of housing and locality. We have argued that these constructed communities developed differing cultures and identities.

The foundation of the welfare state in the postwar period meant that housing became one of the main responsibilities of government. Large sections of working-class people were housed and relocated in new estates or New Towns. During the 1950s and 1960s, economic prosperity and full male employment meant that the model nuclear family upon which the Beveridge Plan had been based made up the 'respectable' working-class tenants of the council estates. Special housing for elderly people was also provided in these areas.

The economic crisis of the late 1970s and the market reforms of the 1980s radically altered the social composition and fragmented the culture of these estates. The rising male unemployment and the decline in relatively well-paid manual work in traditional industries meant the end of the one-occupation communities which had existed since the end of the nineteenth century. The 'right to buy' legislation fragmented council house tenancy. The more desirable houses in attractive areas were bought by sitting tenants and the cessation of any new building by local councils meant that public housing became the site of great social divisions. The 'sink' estates to which the socially and economically marginalized were allocated became notorious and easily identified. In all urban areas, the existence of these 'dangerous places' is well known. Once respectable estates acquired new reputations, people who had moved into these areas in the affluent times were now in older age, surrounded by what appeared to be an alien culture.

The indices of social exclusion (see Chapter 6) are all present in many of these 'no-go areas'. Racial divisions and conflict develop and thrive in areas of shared deprivation and poverty. It is in many of these areas that community nurses practice every day. It is crucial that an understanding of the background, development and culture of the area of practice is gained and applied. Many single young mothers living in these areas articulate their fears of bringing up children surrounded by perceived dangers. The recent incidents involving the 'mob' attacks on suspected paedophiles in Paulsgrove and in South Wales are evidence of the fears of those most vulnerable and also economically powerless. Many older people too living on 'sink' estates live their lives in fear and dread. This situation obviously has outcomes for health and wellbeing.

In tackling health inequalities and engaging in projects to improve health, community nurses must operate with a knowledge of the community and its past as well as present culture and identity. In the chapters which follow, the organisational and cultural changes in professional community-based nursing which are discussed must be set against the necessity for practice to integrate into the culture of a community.

PART II

SELF PORTRAYAL: COMMUNITY NURSES' INVOLVEMENT IN CONSTRUCTING THEIR OWN IDENTITIES

Introduction

The first part of this book has shown how the profession of community nursing, consisting of various groups of nurses, who provide services for both the sick and the well, physically and mentally ill, old and young has evolved as a result of the changing needs of society and the developments in health care policy. We have shown, in previous chapters, how constructions of community nursing have been influenced by the primary motivating imperatives of legitimacy, feasibility and support (Robinson 1982) which incorporate a multitude of other factors such as changing models of health care provision (Baggot 2000), gendered identity considerations (Davies 1995), managerial pragmatism (Hennessy 1995), and the quest on the part of community nurses for professional autonomy and self regulation (Littlewood 1995). These are factors which we have shown to be characterised by Foucault's (1980) theory of power existing within relationships and sites and embodied in the day-to-day practice of the professions. It is suggested that for community nurses these factors may have been powerful constructional forces – tangible forms of policy encountered in the day-to-day experiences of delivering care. Consequently, these factors that were described as governmentality (see Chapter 1) may have contributed much to the way in which community nursing has presented itself to the world at large. Although community nurses did not work within the mechanisms of control designed through governmentality, such as the 'Nightingale' wards of hospitals, they were certainly part of the nineteenth-century's burgeoning discipline of community medicine and public health which Armstrong (1993) described as 'surveillance medicine', and which, throughout the twentieth century, have played an important role in health care developments.

It is the aim of the second part of this book not to comment further on how the concept of governmentality shaped the development of community nursing, but to examine community nurses' struggle to present their own constructions of their roles and the way in which the profession itself has responded to the complicated web of influences constructed by governmentality which has enveloped its beginnings and development and may have made it difficult for community nurses to portray their own identity. This approach is informed by the work of Husserl (1931) who was concerned with the discovery of meanings and essences in knowledge so that essential insights can be gained through the special process of ideation or cognitive interpretation. Because of the fact that on the whole women, and certainly community nurses themselves who were mostly women, are virtually invisible in social history (McClelland 1996), it is difficult to obtain first-hand evidence of their social and economic lives, a fact that was also noted by Hogreffe (1975). In the main, therefore, this section of the book will mostly rely upon other people's interpretations of community nurses experiences, though where possible efforts will be made to convey the thoughts and expressions of nurses themselves.

First, prominent constructions of the profession of community nursing will be explored in order to demonstrate the ambivalences that exist between the concepts of nurses themselves and relevant more powerful others involved in the process of governmentality. Specifically, debate will be centred around whether community nursing is a caring or controlling profession, and whether nurses themselves are able to articulate what they believe to be the real nature of their roles. Evidence of revolutions in nursing will be referred to as the means whereby community nurses themselves attempted to change the course of history and shape their own professional development and status, but it will be seen that these were subjected to governmentality, and the question is raised as to whether nurses will ever shape their own destiny.

Secondly, the shift away from institutionalised models of health care towards primary health care will be explored as a means of illustrating how community nursing has continually metamorphosed in order to meet the demands of changing models of health care provision. It will be shown that although increasing disillusion with their involvement in technological health care, which has been dominated by the medical profession's quest for cure, has awakened in community nurses an interest in the importance of care and maintenance of public health, the difficulties faced by nurses in overcoming the forces of factors mentioned above have often been barriers to the construction of a new identity. It will be argued that, although community nurses might wish to present themselves as a caring profession, policy and systems continue to cast community nurses in a role which could better be described as one of social control of specifically identified patient or client groups, in particular, children, older people and the mentally ill. This observation raises the question of whether the opportunity for the social control of these groups is a positive experience for the people involved and community nurses as their would-be 'carers'?

Thirdly, to illustrate the above argument, the drive to create a modern workforce using new organisation and management strategies will be examined in order to show how managerial forces have continued to have an influence on the construction of community nursing. In particular, it will be argued that the the managerial desire for flexibility in the community nursing workforce has sometimes resulted in marginalisation of nursing care goals, and interference in professional decision-making. The consequences of these developments will be illustrated by means of recent studies which highlight the dilemmas faced by community nurses who are attempting to provide care for people in their own homes. Findings from these studies clearly show how nurses are constantly frustrated in their efforts to provide care, and that, as a result, the public appear to be showing an increasing intolerance of what they interpret as an unsatisfactory service.

Fourthly, the factors which may influence the construction of community nursing in the twenty-first century are addressed. Arguments presented are that the changing environment of health care provision, changing demographic patterns, new technology, alternative health care systems and the availability of human resources may benefit the profession of community nursing. However, for this to happen, it will be necessary for community nurses to play an active role in the development of future services, and to play an active part in the social construction of their profession.

Finally, current ambivalences in the nature of community nursing practice are examined, and the continuing tensions between caring and curing interventions are returned to and further explored. It is argued that for many community nurses a continuing interest and focus on the provision of a technological and medically-orientated service is closely linked to the erroneous belief that this is the means of increasing professional status. Yet, there are many commentators who believe that following such a path will only lead to continued commodification of the profession. It is suggested that the real challenge for community nurses is to show that their caring and controlling roles are relevant and complementary to the public health agenda. To construct a relevant image, it is suggested by prestigious bodies such as the World Health Organisation Study Group (WHO 1984) that, beyond 2000, the way forward for community nurses is to present a pragmatic picture of the aspects of their work which can limit structural causes of ill health, improve public health and facilitate social inclusion of 'hard to help' groups. Ways in which community nurses may attempt to construct a different and new caring image in order to meet the demands of the current public health agenda are explored.

CHAPTER 4

Concepts of Community Nursing

This chapter will explore prevalent constructions of community nursing, and will identify the ambivalences which exist not only in the literature, but also in practitioners' subjective views of their role. Prominent views of the constructs of community nursing are addressed; the community nurse as a carer, and the community nurse as an agent of control, and community nursing as a unified discipline. Reasons for the ambivalences generated by these constructions are discussed. The argument which ensues debates the assumption that community nurses lack the freedom and autonomy to decide for themselves the real nature of their role. Consequently, despite assertions that community nurses are rising to the contemporary challenges of a shift away from the technological thrust of medically-orientated interventions, a phenomenon that has been identified by Dingwall and colleagues, (1988) as the second revolution in nursing, it will be argued that the profession is still beholden to others for the public image of community nursing that emerges. As a consequence, the question of whether community nurses possess sufficient autonomy to articulate and define their own constructs appears to remain unanswered.

A caring profession?

Community nurses have a professional mandate to provide care in the community and to carry out primary health care interventions but, in Radsma's (1994) view, it is often the case that the meanings and functions of the concepts of care and caring presented by nurses are undefined and intangible. Radsma further suggests that, although caring is unquestionably at the root of nursing, caring as the essence of nursing has still to be determined Consequently, the real nature of community nursing may be shrouded in ambivalence and concealed even from nurses themselves. Radsma suggests that beyond a personal meaning of care which nurses apply to their work, few nurses may be aware of what caring from a professional perspective implies. As a result of this conceptual 'gap', social constructions of the role of community nurses may be easily influenced by the constructions of others and the various 'regimes' of truth which have surrounded the discourses on community nursing, past, present and future. Analysis of discourses on care reveal ambivalences in the translation and understanding of this concept therefore it is not suprising that there is some confusion over the exact nature of the caring role of community nurses. However, in order to respond to current pressures of governmentality, it is important that community nurses have a common understanding of the nature of their role. Radsma (1994) asserts that nursing as a profession cannot continue to hide behind the discourse of care without explicit and implicit understanding of what professional caring entails.

Discourses on caring

Dunlop (1986) discovered that the linguistic origins of the term 'care' are related to those of the term 'cure' but, due to class differences in usage of the terms, higher orders of the caring services became involved in cure and lower orders in care. Whilst the meanings of these terms have evolved separately, the distinctions of power remain. Thus the focus of medicine is to cure, whilst nurses have traditionally had a duty to care. It may therefore be the case that nurses' efforts to interpret and theorise the work involved in their care-giving has frequently been subjected to more powerful efforts to translate nursing interpretations into a socially ordered view of the 'natural order' of events. As was shown in Chapter 1, 'powerful' interpretations of governmentality tended to devalue nursing care in favour of developing technological interventions which were the province of the medical profession. It appears, then, that in language discourses, nursing has been perceived as a virtuous duty, an 'unpaid labour of love' particularly for the poor and suffering, such as the old, chronic sick or mentally ill who, according to Reverby (1987), may require an element of social control. Generations of nurses have therefore been subject to the need for acquiescence to medical dominance and an expectation that they would care for groups labelled by society as unresponsive to regimes of cure, a gendered division of labour which was referred to in Chapter 1. Colliere, (1986) suggests that, in an endeavour to rid themselves of the imposed inferiority caused by such aquiesence, nurses have attempted to gain professional prestige but this has been an exercise which has resulted in nurses looking to medicine's use of science, and the submerging of the profession's unique caring skills in curing practices rather than articulation of the theoretical meanings of care-giving. Consequently, the concept of care adopted by nurses has been translated by a number of observers (Davies 1995) into a role of containment complementary to the view of the physician as an agent of social control rather than a supportive role for those who are unable to respond to curative interventions. Although the terms care and caring have traditionally been used by nurses to construct a subjective view of nursing, and to convey to others the inherent worth and value of the profession, much of the history of nursing constructs the profession as an agent of social control (Symonds 1991). This may not be suprising in view of Davies' comments regarding the social constructions of control associated with physicians and the need for the management of poverty, containment of mental illness, medicalisation of child surveillance, containment of epidemics and concerns for the quality and quantity of the population. Dingwall et al. (1988) point out, however, that this is not a construction which maligns community nurses. It should not in any way be seen as pathological or derogatory, nor is it meant to be oppressive or repressive to society. As Dingwall and colleagues explain, properly understood, the term 'care' is merely a pragmatic way of responding to problems which may be faced by particular groups, so that members of such groups can maintain sufficient order to plan and coordinate their daily lives in order to survive (ibid.:24). It is the view of these writers that no society can function without some system of regulation, therefore it should not be too suprising that illness and lack of wellbeing should have been constructed as a form of social deviance. Both are latent disruptive and destabilising forces in society because of their potential to interfere with the performance of normal roles, such as parent, worker, or carer upon which others and society may depend. There is no reason, therefore, why social control should not be seen as an important aspect of care, particularly when it encompasses the support that people require to sustain daily life.

Dingwall and colleagues (1988) suggested, then, that illness or a lack of wellbeing in any section of society attracts the attention of control agencies. For this reason both medicine and nursing have come to be recognised as occupations which are able to define what are acceptable as normal experiences of the human body and what are permissable behaviours as a result of these experiences. Thus, doctors and nurses may define illnesses such as mental disease and distinguish the type of behaviours that can be expected as opposed to those which may be defined as antisocial. These professions therefore offer society the means to return to reality, or to limit the impact of their deviance upon others. It is the view of Dingwall et al. (1988) that, as in many aspects of social life such as education, employment, and policing, the regulation of behaviour has played a part in intensifying control of society in order to support increasing moves towards capitalism and industrialisation. Therefore, the exercise of social control through health care can provide positive experiences of a caring nature as it benefits the public at large, as well as individuals. For example, as was pointed out in Chapter 1, during the nineteenth century the control of diseases and infections such as the cholera outbreaks of 1832 and 1848, as well as typhus typhoid, influenza, scarlet fever, diptheria, smallpox and tuberculosis was essential. These diseases were a real threat to social order, they required the imposition of strict rules of hygiene as a means of imposing discipline on the working classes. Therefore, during the nineteenth and early twentieth century, the control of social behaviour as a means to limit the spread of disease was as important as the control of disease and infection itself.

According to Donzelot (1980), those concerned with social order were inexorably drawn to the regulation of ordinary activities and the development of relationships between the public and the state which would be subtle, sensitive and precisely calculated to wield an iron hand in a velvet glove rather than to punish or forcibly control the deviants (Donzelot 1980). In other words, community nursing like medicine was perceived as an ideal vehicle for both care and social control but, as was suggested in Chapter 1, an identity crisis for community nurses may have been embodied in the dilemma of whether community nursing was a profession for caring educated women or merely a branch of domestic service, in which they were seen merely as adjuncts to male workers who held roles in the 'public' rather than the 'private' domain. Undoubtedly, this debate was particularly contentious in view of the fact that Nightingale herself (1876, quoted in Baly 1986:128 and Dingwall et al. 1988:178), suggested that home nursing required a higher calibre of recruit because of the fact that community nurses were charged with the responsibility of the containment of epidemics and the maintenance of social order. It was not suprising, therefore, that nurses may have reacted to the way in which, on the one hand, governmentality offered them opportunities to care (see Chapter 1) and, on the other hand, these opportunities were thwarted by prevalent social controls such as gender constraints. It appears, then, that the important contributions made by community nurses to health and social care may have been subjugated by the constraints of social norms, or at least they were hidden from view, as a result of gendered discourses. As was seen in Chapter 1, community nurses may have been important agents of social control but they also were guides, philosophers and friends to whole neighbourhoods (Stocks 1960:16).

Revolutions in community nursing

At the beginning of the nineteenth century, there was a period of rapid change and social upheaval which disrupted social cohesion, and community nursing underwent what has been described by Dingwall and colleagues (1988:22) as its first revolution, a phrase which describes the evolution of a new style of nursing in response to a new style of medicine based on experimental interventions and scientific research. As it developed, nursing became an important agent of social control (p. 26), a process which has already been described in Chapter 1 and which Donzelot (1980:55–8) describes as a way to control sections of the population without coercion by the state. Far from being an intrusive action, Donzelot (1980), agreeing with Dingwall et al. (ibid.) describes the concept of social control as a style of public intervention which provides assistance, defined as economic aid for the needy, and medical hygienism, interventions which were essential for the control of poverty and disease as well as public health (see Chapter 1). This definition of social control incorporated a model of respectable living for those who were physically or morally ill equipped to enjoy a decent life style. In Donzelot's view, although emphasis was placed on the importance of social control, this was really a kind of social support which placed community nurses in the 'front line' of public health developments. In practice, it led to the development of community nursing services which organised middle- and upper-class women to visit the homes of the poor in order to further the Christian ideals of self discipline, sobriety and domestic economy, and to provide home nursing, Far from being oppressive, Donzelot suggests that this first revolution in nursing brought about an important alliance between women and the state. The interventions provided by community nurses, particularly district nurses and health visitors in the home, and school and factory (as described in Chapter 1) provided support and empowerment for women and children particularly in conditions of sheer grinding poverty which the state did little to assuage (Pember Reeves 1913). In contrast, feminist historians have emphasised that the process of social control was introduced into nursing in order to control the working classes. Donzelot (1980) suggests that this is not strictly true, a fact supported in Chapter 1, where it was recognised that the services described had a capacity to mediate the grievances of groups which may have been constructed as excluded from the nation by virtue of their needs or perceived deficiencies. It is the view of Donzelot that in exchange for community nurses accepting a role as bearers of social discipline, the primary initial role of community nurses was to provide a form of social support and to educate the population to deal with the many factors that disrupt health and wellbeing.

However, obfuscation of liberal interpretations of the meaning of the term social control means that a view emerged that community nurses functioned as an 'inspectorate' to maintain social order. This is a view that remains prevalent (Davies 1988), and it is suggested that it has emerged from the efforts on the part of nursing to improve the status of the profession by emulating medicine, and has been sustained as a result of interpreting caring functions through the paradigms of interventions aimed at curing the sick and modifying behaviour. Though, as Dingwall (1982:340) points out, this is a construct which may have become prevalent as a result of middle-class health visitors being licensed to exercise their authority in improving health and wellbeing. This authority involved creating a balance between libertarian values and enforcement in the lives of uneducated working-class women.

Nearly two centuries after the first 'revolution', nursing is facing a second revolution which is said to have been been promoted by dissatisfaction with current models of health care (European Conference on Nursing (ECN) 1988). Such dissatisfactions are said (ECN 1988) to have been fuelled by nurses appreciation of the shift away from biomedical models of care. The need for emphasis on health promotion and prevention in an effort to deal with issues of cost and efficiency, the ageing population and declining birth rates of the western world, increases in infectious and chronic illness, mental and social problems, and the wider use of advanced technology, have been signalled repeatedly by the World Health Organisation (WHO) since the International Conference of Alma Ata in 1978. Whereas both of the so-called revolutions in nursing could be viewed merely as a perceived response to dissatisfaction with services offered, in contrast to the first revolution which Dingwall and colleagues (1988) saw as being directed by the profession of medicine, the second revolution has been influenced by nurses themselves. This 'second revolution' has been instigated by nurses from thirty-two member states of the WHO's European Region in response to Primary Health Care (PHC) strategy (Morrow 1988). In the UK, the revolutionary movement has also been supported by a number of government and professional reports (Symonds and Kelly 1998) which have challenged the nursing profession to identify the ways in which they can contribute to the shift towards primary health and community care. Differences in the driving forces behind these 'revolutions' in nursing appear to be characterised by the extent of professional autonomy that nurses have developed over time to articulate the preferred nature of their interventions. Autonomy is characterised by events such as the European Conference on Nursing (1988) which claimed that nursing has an important role to play in primary health care, and that nursing practice is changing to meet society's evolving needs. Yet, the question of whether nursing has a more prominent role and autonomy in national health plans as a result of this so-called second revolution is not debated. Although recommendations for the development of nursing services emphasise the role of the community nurse in health rather than disease and care rather than cure, the profession itself has been slow to articulate how patterns of care should change. This so-called revolution on the part of nurses makes it more important than ever that community nurses are able to articulate what they mean by care. Commentators on the profession of nursing, such as Hyde (1995), suggest that, on the whole, it still appears to be dominated by hospital-style interventions and practice. This means that the scope of nursing practice may be more technological than care focused and is more likely to be based on medical rather than social interventions. Thus, community nursing appears to be focused more at the sharp end of front-line intervention than at the interface of social and health care where needs are more diverse, and is complicated by the requirements of providing ongoing care in the less dramatic settings of the community. As a result, nursing care appears to be less focused on public health needs, and health care services may be hampered by the fact that insufficient account is taken of demographic and epidemiological trends, social and physical environments, lifestyles, cultural values and economic choices, and their effects on health. If these factors are considered, as is currently the recommendation of the NHS Plan (DoH 2000), care delivered by community nurses could be facilitated through the provision of economic aid, hygienism and social support to excluded groups. In the absence of such public-health nursing interventions, it may be the case, that the social construction of the community nursing profession, as one which enables people to achieve a maximum potential of health and wellbeing, will remain weak. Consequently, nursing potential may be lost if nurses themselves persist in a reluctance to define what they mean by care, and to distinguish their understanding of the term 'social control' as a means of providing caring social support rather than a function to ensure social order. However, this may not be a simple task for, as Hyde (1995) has pointed out, a number of different groups of nurses constitute the profession of community nursing, and, this being the case, it is possible that each group might hold a different interpretation of what the concepts of 'care' and 'caring' mean for them.

Diversity in community nursing

Hyde (1995) suggested that the umbrella term 'community nursing' seems to imply that those involved in the profession have common characteristics, similar functions and are part of a coordinated network. The United Kingdom Central Council for Nursing Midwifery and Health Visiting (UKCC), now the Nursing and Midwifery Council (2002), in a paper entitled 'The Future of Professional Practice, constructed community nursing in this way – The Council's Standards for Education and Practice Following Registration (UKCC 1994) stated that there was a 'new discipline of community health care nursing' a statement which implied a common ideological base and identity for all eight branches of community nursing. This is a strategy highlighted in the first section of this book as a move to implement skill-mix and thereby potentially increase flexibility. However, as Hyde (1995) points out, the professional focus of community nursing is diverse and its characteristics, functions, practices and networks vary in accordance with what McMurray (1990:10) describes as a concept of practice, that is whether the focus of practice is on conservation of health, prevention of harmful changes, restoration to optimal levels of health following illness, or the amelioration of illness and its effects. This is a view which echoes that of Hyde (1995) in that there is no support for the concept of community nursing being a unified discipline, or indeed a discipline at all. As Hyde, quoting Butterworth (1988:36) points out, community nurses can be grouped into eight different specialties; district nursing, health visiting, community psychiatric nursing, community mental handicap nursing, school nursing, occupational health nursing, practice nursing and community midwives and each of these specialties may hold a different perception of the role of a community nurse. Indeed, some of these groups may even refute the title of community nurse. Midwives, for example, are not necessarily nurses, and in the past neither were health visitors (see Chapter 1). Opportunities for direct entry to the profession mean that eventually the proportion of midwives who are also nurses may markedly decrease. The Winterton Report (DoH 1993) certainly demonstrated that midwives wish to be recognised as a profession that is independent from nursing. Reviews of Health Visiting (UKCC 2001, Clark et al. 2000) have also shown that health visitors have an unique role which differs markedly from nursing. Thus, it can be seen that the idea of there being one construction of community nursing may be completely without foundation, as not only are there different specialties of community nursing, and different recipients of care, but the foci of care may also differ. Whereas the majority of community nurses may provide care to individuals, some groups such as health visitors, occupational health nurses and school nurses must of necessity provide care for communities (NAfW 2000), for example, in schools, defined geographical areas, workplaces or communities. These groups focus on the health of populations which become the 'client', and therefore practise public health intervention rather than individual clinical care. These considerations pose the question of whether the social constructions of 'care' and 'caring' are the same for all branches of community nursing, and whether it is suprising that there is no consensus on the nature of community nursing care. Watson (1984) suggested that the construction of the role of community nurses should be influenced by the way in which individual groups of nurses practice, and not by a concern to mould community nurses into a flexible commodity merely to comply with shifts in policy strategy or to meet the agendas of more powerful groups involved in the delivery of community care services. It might therefore be the case that only some groups of community nurses are preoccupied with the notions of care, whilst others prefer to direct their energies into developing skills of a technological and curing nature. If this is the case, diversity should be valued and all community nurses should be given equal opportunities to articulate the real nature of their role.

Exploding the myth of the concept of the generic community nurse

Questioning whether the concept of the community nurse is appropriate to convey the caring functions of all branches of the profession, Hyde (1995) suggests that the single label is misleading and confusing. In her view, the amalgamation of all branches of community nursing into one unified group might have the same effect as suggesting that hospital nursing and community nursing are one and the same thing, and that all are involved in delivering the same model of care. According to Hyde (1995:2), the popular concept of the 'community nurse' has been shaped by mistaken beliefs that;

> community nursing is the same as hospital nursing: skills are simply transferred to a different setting,
>
> community nursing is peripheral to the centrality of hospital nursing,
>
> community nursing is primarily about visiting the sick,

and that

> 'all community nurses share an unified vision of the nature of care'.

Commenting on the fact that portrayals of the role of community nurses commonly seen in the media are those of a clinical nurse, Hyde (1995) recognises that this construction of community nursing may also be perpetuated by those community nurses who resist political and professional pressures to adopt a health-orientated approach to care. Instead, they opt to fulfill the traditional nurse role and preserve familiar territory by preferring to excercise skills more suited to the 'sharp' end of care, thus ensuring compliance with technological intervention rather that a concern with public health. Thus, the kind of nursing interventions which provide care and support through the exercise of social control are less obvious and inadequately valued. For this reason, it is important to identify current influences on the construction of the concept of community nursing and to discuss how these may help the various groups which constitute the profession to play a more prominent role in shaping their futures, and make the value of the caring role more explicit. The shift from institutional care, and the emphasis on primary health care and care in the community signalled by the NHS and Community Care Act (DoH 1990) combined to provide an important challenge to community nurses in respect of determining whether community nursing can be constructed as a controlling or an enabling profession by the people that it serves.

Primary health care and community care

Macdonald (1992:9) defined Primary health care (PHC) as an approach to the provision of health care through a partnership between health, other professionals and the community, to promote health and meet the needs of the majority of the population, as well as provide a system of treatment and curative care. According to Macdonald (ibid.) this new model of health care constitutes a major revolution in the pattern of health care delivery as, up until now, most societies have employed a model of health care which has mainly focused on curative care based in institutions and governed by the medical profession. However, he suggests that new directions are certainly needed in the provision of health care services as health systems in most countries are experiencing difficult times, and serious questions are being asked about their effectiveness and appropriateness. It is Macdonald's view that a completely new kind of health care system is needed and that the blueprint for such a system was laid out at the International Conference of Alma Ata in 1978, convened by the World Health Organisation (WHO) and the United Nations International Conference (UNICEF) (WHO 1986). At this conference, the failure of 'western medicine' to address many of the basic health needs of developing countries was noted, and guidelines for new ways of thinking about and planning health care systems were identified. These guidelines, in Macdonald's view, constitute a revolutionary 'Trojan horse' for medical practice. It is his belief that the proposed revolution in health care can be likened to the Greek legend in which the people of Troy admitted into their walled city a wooden horse which unknown to them contained their enemy the Greeks. Whilst the city of Troy slept, the Greeks emerged from the horse and opened the gates of the city to their invading army, which overcame the Trojans, and cleared the way for the installation of a new regime. Given that this analogy has some relevance to changing patterns of health care delivery, the question of its immediate relevance to the social construction of the profession of community nursing is raised. If nurses who work in community settings can provide answers to the questions of what primary health care and community care mean to them, and the nature of care they can contribute to this evolutionary development, it might be possible for them to 'shake off' the medical domination which has stifled their role development in the past. At the European Conference on Nursing in Vienna (1988), nurses claimed to have a major role to play in new developments in health care. They identified the need for a skilful and dedicated health professional, a generalist nurse, a flexible worker whose work would involve the main themes of the 'Health for All' movement (WHO 1986). It was identified that such a nurse would live in the community and maintain regular contact with individuals and families in their homes, schools and workplaces, but little consideration appears to have been given to how 'nursing could be strengthened to bring health into every area of people's lives and work. Nor to how generic nurses might provide expertise in a broad range of health care and functions', thereby exercising a model of care which equates with Dingwall et al.'s (1988) and Donzelot's (1980) interpretations of social control as a form of public health intervention.

It would therefore appear that in the enthusiasm to embrace a new concept of care provision, namely primary public health, and to expand the caring aspect of their roles, nurses may have given little thought to the diverse needs of society and the range and spectrum of care and cure needed to fulfill a primary health-care function. Confusion over the very different concepts of primary health care and primary medical care, and the different range of social and medical interventions involved in these processes Macdonald (1998), may have prevented nurses from appreciating that community health nursing consists of a wide range of practice and different philosophies regarding the nature of health, healing and care (Aggleton 1990). Far from being a generalist activity, the breadth of community practice covers preventive, promotive, rehabilitative and ameliorative activities. It is difficult to see how all of these functions can be embraced by a generalist nurse who would presumably replace all of the current branches of community nursing. This was a fact recognised by McMurray (1990:122) who affirmed that the practice of community health nursing is as diverse as the clients and settings it serves. In her view 'community nurses should define nursing practice according to their commitment to primary health care with its associated concepts and values'. Failure to recognise that the concept of PHC is a collaborative approach towards the promotion of health and wellbeing and to meeting the needs of all people, as well as the provision of a system of treatment and curative care, may well have hampered the progress of development of community nursing to establish itself as a caring and empowering profession. As Hyde (1995), suggests, the umbrella term 'community nurse' masks the divergence of caring activity carried out by community nurses and promotes the concept that the only differences in the nature of the various professional groups involved in community nursing is the setting in which they work, or the age and diagnosis of the people with whom they come in contact. Why then has this situation arisen? One explanation might be that the distinction made between medical and social interpretations of health care since the Alma Ata agreement has disguised from nurses the fact that, although medically-orientated interventions are important, they are not paramount, and that revolutions in health care call for evolutionary changes in the construction of the focus of community nursing interventions. Therefore, a collaborative form of care provision spanning the whole range of caring interventions from prevention to amelioration may be more empowering for communities than individual forms of control.

Baggott (2000) suggests that the current changes in respect of a new revolution in health care provision have been evolutionary and that developments can be traced from the early days of public health – and the time that Dingwall and colleagues (1988) describe as the first revolution in nursing. Thus, community nursing has always had to metamorphose to meet changing needs, and the pressures of governmentality. As was seen in Chapter 1, community nurses have subsequently been influenced through the transfer of Poor Law systems to National Health Insurance Schemes; the setting up of a network of local authority community health services such as midwifery, district nursing and health visiting services that worked closely with voluntary associations; the school medical service which after 1912 moved beyond inspection and diagnosis to the development of school nursing, dental and opthalmic services; extension of child and maternal services from 1918; and the growth of local authorities during the 1920s and 30s which culminated in the Poor Law hospitals being brought under the control of Health Committees following the 1929 Local Government Act; and the transfer of responsibility for certain services such as maternity and child welfare, tuberculosis management, immunisation services, blind people and those with mental deficiency to the local authorities. These developments paved the way for a divide in the provision of public health and hospital care, and thus a divide in the focus of nursing interventions. Slowly, over time, the profession of nursing appears to have been primarily channelled into focusing its attention on intervention rather than on activities that prevent disease and illness, to medical rather than social forms of care. It may therefore be unrealistic to expect that current PHC and public health policy should result in an immediate appreciation of the fact that medical and social types of intervention require different skills. The mere transference of nursing skills into community settings is insufficient to equip community nurses with the broad range of competencies that they require to ensure public health (Llewellyn and Trent 1987:2). Therefore, although community nurses may be frustrated in their attempts to meet the requirements of emerging policy by the failure of their leaders to appreciate that diverse and contrary philosophies cannot be put together to 'create' a new discipline (Hyde 1995:23), the failure of nurses themselves to determine the real nature of caring in community settings may mean that nurses have missed opportunities to take a lead in the facilitation of primary health and community services that provide supportive care to client groups and improve the public health through inclusion of disadvantaged groups in healthful activity.

Revival in public health services can be traced to a number of events, since the 1970s there have been criticisms of the role of medicine in health care, rising costs and failures in public health. Cochrane (1971), for example, noted the need for a rigorous evaluation of health services, and McKeown (1976) argued that modern medicine was too individualised and disease orientated to recognise the wider social, economic and environmental influences on health, contending that the contribution of medicine to the decline of disease was exaggerated. To support his thesis, McKeown showed how, as a result of improved nutrition and rising standards of living, infectious diseases such as measles, whooping cough and tuberculosis had declined well before the advent of immunisation and medical treatment. It was also his view that reductions in mortality and morbidity since the late nineteenth century were the result of improved hygiene, and that the major causes of ill health in today's society such as cancer, heart diseases and respiratory disease which result from individual behaviour and environmental factors can be prevented. Therefore, in his view, excessive reliance on medicine has resulted in an inadequate and belated response to the disease process. Although McKeown's thesis has been criticised on several counts (Sagan 1987:102, Bunker et al. 1994, Bynum 1994), it serves to highlight the wider causes of ill health which can be prevented by more caring interventions based on the social control of public health. In Baggott's (2000) view, McKeown's thesis fuels a debate on the way in which health care services are resourced, and the need for broader health care strategies to promote health and prevent disease. This debate came to a head when, in 1988, the Chief Medical Officer Donald Acheson conducted an inquiry into the state of public health (Cm289 1988) and reported that it was in a state of crisis. In 1991, the Conservative Government led by John Major published a Green Paper, *The Health of the Nation* (Cmd523 1991) in which the aims of 'adding years to life, adding life to years', increasing life expectancy and reducing premature death were identified. Although, following consultation on this document, a White Paper (Cm. 1986, 1992) identified targets for reduction of the incidence of morbidity and mortality, placed the notions of preventive health care and health improvement firmly on the agenda, and increased awareness of the need for health promotion (Baggot 2000), doctors and the majority of nurses were slow to take up the public health challenge. The Faculty of Public Health Medicine (1991) noted that this shortfall occurred despite the fact that the extent of the public health challenge merely suggested targets for health promotion which reflected a medical rather than a social perspective of health (Radical Statistics Health Group 1991), and were disease rather than health orientated. What clearly emerged from this situation was a recognition that individual pathology rather than a concern for socio-economic causes of ill health was the main concern of doctors and nurses. Critics of the ability of the strategy to meet public health needs challenged the use of health gain targets, identified by the strategy documents on the grounds that they downgraded health problems to the status of quantifiable measurements (Baum and Saunders 1988). It was the view of these critics that, as health problems were often too difficult to quantify because of their complex nature, a mere form of selective primary health care characterised by health gain targets was more acceptable to doctors and the majority of nurses. But in no way did this approach meet the health needs of the population. In the main, only a minority of nurses, mostly health visitors, took a more comprehensive view of the nature of health care needed but they were silenced by technocrats, and found it difficult to practise even a modified and medicalised version of primary health care (Symonds and Kelly 1998). On the whole, the majority of nurses like their medical counterparts were only prepared to pay lip service to primary health care developments as they had little inclination to explore the real nature of health care problems and the real nature of caring in community settings.

Given the confusion which still appears to exist over the concept of primary health care, it may not be suprising that community nurses are still unclear as to what is required of them in terms of their contribution to the evolutionary developments in health care services, and the caring role that they should play in bringing about a second revolution in the profession. In addition to the conceptual confusion that nurses have had to confront as a result of medical and managerial interpretations of primary health care strategy, the monopoly of community nurses in the provision of care in the community has been further disrupted by the introduction of the NHS and Community Care Act (1990). Transference of the responsibility for the organisation of community care to local authorities (McCarthy 1989) has meant that shortages of nursing resources have increased concerns over the quality of caring provided by nurses. To add to this problem, cost limitation has been conveniently masked by increasing use of informal and ancillary care and eloquent discourses on the advantages of a 'mixed economy of care' which have sent out messages that social care is no longer a concern of community nurses. Similarly, constraints on the public health focus of health visiting practice (Kelly et al. 1998) have signalled that medical interventions of care are more important than social care. Together then, interpretations of the discourses of community care and primary health care may have constrained the independence and autonomy of community nurses to determine for themselves the effects of evolutionary progress on desirable construction of community nursing. In order to preserve the legitimacy of their professional status, it has been suggested by Ackroyd (1998) that community nurses have had to conform to efforts to increase the flexibility of their resource by acceding to others' interpretations of how they can best serve current agendas of care. Despite the fact that for the last three decades a proliferation of documents relating to the professional development of nursing have emphasised the importance of role definition, it would appear that specific roles for community nurses, based upon a particular concept of care, and specific portrayals of community nursing as a profession intent on enabling and empowering the public have yet to emerge (Kelly 1998). Although improved educational opportunities (UKCC 1986, 1992 and 1994) have increased the academic status of community nurses, a blurring of community nurse roles, for the purpose of conforming to prevalent constructions of primary health and community care concepts, appears to have focused attention on the maintenance of social order amongst specific care groups rather than on the specific type of care and social support that should be delivered to these groups and the public at large by different branches of community nursing, in order to enhance social control and inclusion. Thus, it is the view of Baumgart (1998) that, if community nurses are to enhance their image as professional carers and uphold their commitment to directing evolutionary change, 'it must be nurses that define nursing practice according to their commitment to primary health and community care, with its associated concepts and values' and not the need to maintain social order amongst specific care groups. Taking this view, McMurray suggests that, far from amalgamating interventions and blurring roles through the adoption of a shared 'title', community nursing should celebrate the fact that its practice is as diverse as the clients and settings that it serves. Oda (1985) suggested that this could be achieved by different branches of community nurses prioritising their caring activities and articulating their role limits so that their caring service is manageable, visible, definable and indispensable.

Barriers to the construction of a new concept of community nursing which incorporates care and social control

Currently, the conceptual confusion over whether community nursing can be seen as a unified discipline (Hyde 1995) concerned more with curing than caring is no doubt affected by the conceptual confusion over the concept of Primary Health Care (PHC). Macdonald (1998) pointed out that the debate over different forms of PHC has had a considerable impact on the forms which health services have taken. Debates on the merits of 'selective' or 'comprehensive' forms of PHC demonstrate, in Macdonald's view, the power of the medical profession in shaping health services provided in community settings. The Alma Ata Conference of 1979 provided the world with a 'strong' vision of comprehensive PHC, which demonstrated how various sectors such as agriculture, environmental health and education played as important a role as the medical profession in controlling the many determinants of health which exist in addition to heredity, physiology and infection as factors which cause ill health, and are amenable to medical intervention. This comprehensive view of PHC embraces the notion that people's participation in health care planning is a crucial dimension of health services. Similarly, the comprehensive approach acknowledges the importance of ensuring that justice and equity are essential components of health care if the effects of poverty and deprivation upon health status are to be reduced. Selective PHC supporters on the other hand take the view that limited resources for health care dictate that interventions must be carefully selected and targeted onto the 'most deserving' groups within the population. Usually these are groups that require to be controlled because of their inability to care for themselves, such as the elderly, mentally ill, and mentally handicapped women and children, whose health needs can be temporarily alleviated by the use of low cost interventions. Warren (1988:891) suggested that selective PHC could be the best means of improving the health of the greatest number of people but, Banerji (1984) drew attention to the political dimensions of such an argument by suggesting that moves from 'strong' to 'weak' versions of PHC are characterised by appropriate technico-medical interventions delivered to the public by health workers who are less qualified than doctors. This is a process which may mask the general implications of the priority decisions and obscure the need for political and social reform to remove structural barriers to health. According to this view, seemingly praiseworthy health programmes which stress the value of short-term technical interventions serve the interests of those who oppose social change for the inclusion of excluded groups into the main stream of society. It is into this argument that nurses have been drawn through their failure to define the real nature of care, and their acquiescence to accept a generalist role in community health care so that their activities can be focused on low-cost technico-medical interventions employed in selective health care strategies such as *The Health of The Nation* health gain targets (DoH 1991). Thus, over the last decade, community nurse practice has been subjected to discourses of 'effectiveness' and forced to provide a form of commodified care which Macdonald (1992) describes as consisting of a package of technical interventions, the outcomes of which can be easily measured. According to Macdonald, this approach is not 'a people empowering process' but a mere extension of low-cost medical services, which in community settings means that the need for services is 'diagnosed' on the basis of professional opinions of what is wrong with a population, and the prescription for intervention follows. For example, the programme for the control of athsma and the programme for the control of influenza in the elderly population (DoH 1992) illustrate how interventions may merely provide a 'quick fix' rather than deal with the underlying causes of ill health. Thus, far from involving community nurses in the empowerment of people and communities, such programmes have served to increase the medicalisation of nursing interventions, have curtailed public health activity and modified the real nature of caring interventions. Thus, it is concluded that in their effort to embrace the impetus for a shift away from medical models of care, provided by the Alma Ata Declaration, nurses may have been led into a blind alley where they find themselves more responsible for low-'tech' medical interventions which reduce the cost of health care, than public health strategies designed to care for people and empower disadvantaged sections of the community.

Conclusion

This chapter has shown how, since the beginning of the nineteenth century, community nurses through governmentality have been required to conform to prevalent discourses and power systems. In conforming, nurses have been offered the opportunity to express the caring nature of the role afforded them in ensuring social control. However, the importance of this role has often been rejected or overlooked as a result of pressures from more powerful groups to conform with traditional female roles and thereby medical orientations of care. Recent shifts towards care in the community and primary health care have challenged nurses to construct a new identity for themselves. This involves becoming empowerers of people disadvantaged by society, and providers of a form of care and social intervention which, although it might be described as social control, is best interpreted as a desirable form of social support, rather than the maintenance of social order. It has been shown, however, that the implementation of community services over the past decade, governed by public sector management may have compromised the development of community nursing services. Discourses relating to various models of PHC delivery may have been responsible for curtailing the caring activity of community nurses and ensuring that their activity is more medically than socially orientated. The following chapter will discuss this speculative assumption in greater depth.

CHAPTER 5

Constructions of Community Nursing Roles

Introduction

In this chapter, various influences which have led to current constructions of community nursing roles are examined and the efforts of community nurses themselves to build a new identity are explored. As was seen in Chapter 2, throughout most of the twentieth century, there was a growing belief that ill health could be prevented by the amelioration of risk, and that people had a personal responsibility for risk limitation. Movement away from concerns about infectious disease (Baggot 2000) meant that there was a hiatus in linkages between diseases of the body and mind with social spaces. This denial of the fact that people sharing a geographical or socio-economic space were often likely to be prone to specific forms of ill health or dysfunctional social behaviour was, in many ways, reminiscent of how the French philosopher and mathematician, Descartes, in his thesis *Trait de l'homme (1662)* quoted in Porter (1999:217) dismissed any relationship between body and mind. It is therefore argued that, as the reponsibility for health became more personalised, the role of community nurses became increasingly influenced by medical orientations of health care. This was almost inevitable in the light of the fact that the type of health services adopted in Britain were based upon access to medical expertise rather than a collectivist public health approach. This was a situation which was exacerbated following the introduction of the NHS in 1948 when health care became centered in the public sphere of hospitals and institutions, and all nurses by virtue of a medically-orientated training were likely to become blinkered from public disease and squalor by the perceived glamour or drama of 'front-line' care. Whilst hospital nurses benefitted from the rapid technological revolution in health care, the increasing costs in health care noted by the Guillebaud Committee 1953 (MoH 1956) were already prompting reconsiderations about the most economical settings for health care. However, the NHS continued to be primarily a hospital service and hospital nurses continued to increase their technological skills, whilst at the same time throughout the 1960s and 1970s community nurses were aware of the clouds gathering on the horizon as the result of the increasingly apparent inadequacies of the welfare state. As was seen in Chapter 2, these inadequacies were catalogued by researchers like Abel Smith and Townsend (1965), and by television producers in programmes such as *Cathy come Home* (1966), a documentary on the plight of the homeless, but care and support offered in such circumstances by community nurses went unrecognised as the spotlight of governmentality became increasingly focused on streamlining nursing to fit the plans for large 'high tech' hospitals (see Chapter 2). There can be no doubt that during this period there was an increasing emphasis on hospital nursing whilst community nurses had a subordinate role, and their voice was not heard.

This chapter will commence at the point in the 1960s where legislation was introduced for the sole purpose of streamlining nursing, and the effects of legislation upon community nurses will be discussed. As the discussion progresses further, effects of governmentality on the roles of community nurses will be explored and nursing responses examined. A consideration of current constructions of community nursing and the challenges posed by new perceptions of the concept of health and the need for community development will bring the chapter to a close.

Community nursing roles

Chapter 2 has clearly shown how the profession of community nursing may have been hampered by pressures on the profession to comply with policy, managerial pragmatism, the influence of the medical profession, issues related to gendered identity, public expectations, and a failure of the community nursing profession to communicate the broad spectrum of unrecognised health determinants that were slowly undermining the nation's health and wellbeing, and how fragmentation of health and social care was disadvantaging and excluding certain groups of people from their rights as citizens to receive care. The effect of these factors is examined in greater depth in the following sections.

Influences of government policy

The willingness of the nursing profession to comply with and be 'shaped' by government policy is evidenced in much of its history (see Chapters 1 and 2). As a result, all branches of community nursing experienced contraction of the social aspect of their caring roles, following the introduction of the NHS. Chapter 2 describes how the role of district nurses became narrowed when an emphasis was placed on the need for a medical health service in the community and the social aspect of their role was diverted to other occupations. As a result, district nursing became largely a 'hidden occupation' marginal to the direction of technological advancement which was determining the 'state of the art' in hospital care. As a result, the scope of practice of district nurses was narrowed and their caring interventions became confined to the elderly sick in their own homes whilst their responsibilities for social care and education of families was placed elsewhere. Connections between health visitors and social care also became dislocated, though perhaps not to the same extent as was the case for distrct nurses. In this instance, there was a 'pull and push' effect, as on the one hand health visitors were drawn into the developing area of community medicine whilst on the other hand they were still expected to carry out the functions specified in the Jameson Report (MoH 1956a), namely, health education, the provision of social advice, collaboration with other workers (such as GPs and social workers, particularly in the field of child protection and child care). However, the dislocation of health visitors from their prominent role in public health gradually came to mean that the profession suffered from a form of 'anomie'. They did not belong totally in either the health or the social sphere, a situation which was eventually to lead almost to their disenfranchisement from the nursing profession.

Following the Education Act of 1944, school nursing enjoyed a period of development (see Chapter 2) where they were expected to participate in the organisation and delivery of school medical services and provide health education especially for girls. Gradually, however, the emergence of the 'market' in health care saw a decline in the numbers of school nurses. A similar fate applied to occupational health nurses who, although following the institution of the NHS, enjoyed an expansion in their services as a result of the nationalisation of industries, with industrial decline, they too decreased in numbers and authority (Charley 1978). In contrast to the above groups, mental health nursing did not develop as a branch of community nursing until the middle of the 1970s, but for some time to come it remained very much in the shadow of medical interventions for the mentally ill. Thus, it can be seen that the increased emphasis on the importance of medical services meant that the social role of community nurses was seriously eroded to the extent that eventually they came to work mostly with groups suffering from incurable disorders such as the chronic sick and the old, and those sections of the community who were deemed to need surveillance such as mothers and young children.

Restructuring and its effects on nursing roles

The changes outlined above did not take place in a vacuum, as can be seen from Chapter 2 they reflected the broader transformations taking place in the wider society, particularly changes in the location and methods of delivering health care. As Nettleton (1995:214) observes, these changes were characterised in the literature by shifts from modernism to post or late modernism at one level and from Fordism to post-Fordism at the level of the economy. As Nettleton explains, these terms refer to the changes that started in the 1970s when in relation to welfare there was a shift from mass universal needs being met by monolithic, paternalistic, professionally-led bureacracies to a situation of welfare pluralism. Such social transformations became evident in the restructuring of the nursing profession, in its withdrawal from the community and public health, and the gradual expansion in local authority social care and the voluntary sector (see Chapter 2) to take its place.

Dingwall and colleagues (1998) show how, in the 1940s, the Wood Committee, and in the 1970s, the Briggs Committee (MoH 1947, HMSO 1972) imposed changes on the nursing professions in the guise of a need for structural change in the delivery of health care (also discussed in Chapter 2). The continuing compliance of the profession with policy was demonstrated by its acceptance of the passage of the Nurses, Midwives and Health Visitors' Act (1979) which rejected the professions' wish for autonomous practice in favour of low-cost administrative reform. Similarly following the 'Harding Report' (SMAC and SNMAC 1981) which provided community nurses with an opportunity for integrated cooperation with staff from different professional disciplines, they were subjected to a form of organisation which reconciled the need for teamwork with the need to provide adequate nursing services along the lines of a medical model. As a result, fragmentation of care resulted (see Chapter 2). Although, consequently, the recommendations of the Cumberlege Report (DHSS 1986) recognised an increasingly important role for community nurses, not just in the treatment room, but in screening procedures, health education, preventive programmes, and as a first point of contact for young and older people, these recommendations were rejected by the government who were reluctant to act on the findings of the report because of doctors' views that it was 'tampering with the territory of the medical profession'. Yet, paradoxically, at the same time there was government sympathy for the medical professions' arguments for an ancillary payments scheme to allow the employment of practice nurses to relieve them of preventive care tasks. Fatchett (1994:216) comments on how the rejection of this report did community nursing a great disservice and led to its diminution in the field of community care and public health.

The influence of management on the roles of community nurses

The introduction of general management in the mid 1980s, as a result of the Griffiths inquiry into NHS Management (DHSS 1983), provided yet another phase in the contest between managerial and professional versions of nursing. Yet again the 'frontier of control' was shifted from professional community nurses to managers, and health service managers became increasingly involved in decisions over the nature of community nursing practice. This resulted in discourses on 'flexibility' which served to disguise the restructuring of community nursing teams to suit the professional focus and needs of 'fundholding' general practitioners rather than the specialist focus of the various groups of community nurses (Symonds and Kelly 1998). From 1987 onwards, the government's active stance towards 'primary care' increased, the discourse, however, omitted the word health from the equation thus indicating that there was more interest in the control of resources and provision than the philosophical meaning embraced by the philosophy of PHC forwarded by the WHO (1978). The White Paper, *Promoting Better Health* (DHSS 1987), clearly presented an emphasis on 'new managerialism' and placed the lead for primary care with the GP thereby making primary health care synonymous with 'personal medical services' rather than 'Health for All'.

As a result of these developments, the work of many community nurses such as health visitors, school nurses and district nurses that was centred on a more expanded notion of primary health care and social intervention became increasingly invisible. It would appear that the more out of step community practice was with medical interventions the more its legitimacy seemed to decrease. Thus, health visitors and school nurses, in particular, may have become valued only for the extent to which they could maintain social order among aberrant populations such as child abusers, ineffective parents, one-parent families, the elderly, pregnant teenagers, young drug abusers and children with problem behaviours. The only apparent commodity that a health visitor might offer a GP was clinic work, as it helped to fill a vital function of the GP contract (DoH 1989), that is surveillance and immunisation of the under fives population. As a result, the public health focus of health visiting and school nursing became seriously curtailed. District nurses also suffered as a result of the NHS and Community Care Act (DoH 1990), as changes in the role of local authorities to 'purchasers' rather than 'providers' of services, meant that district nurses found their caring role was increasingly usurped by personnel working in the independent or local authority sector. To contain cost, boundaries were redefined between health and social, and formal and informal care providers, thus the nature of district nursing care was transformed to technical intervention rather than supportive nurturing. Consequently, through the advent of new managerialism and the changes initiated in health and social care, as a result of the NHS and Community Care Act (ibid.), the nature of caring and what could be legitimately purchased as 'health care' became narrower. Similarly, the therapeutic aspects of mental health nursing were reduced in many instances to custody and control.

According to Ackroyd (1998) the effects of the 'management revolution' have been felt disproportionately by nurses, although the medical profession has not escaped lightly (Symonds and Kelly 1998). In Ackroyd's opinion, nurses should not have been surprised at the way in which their roles were reconstructed because of the fact that the provision of nursing services is a large component of the cost of health care. Despite the fact that nurses are low paid, Ackroyd showed that, in 1996, their salaries cost the NHS £8 billion, and therefore he suggested that it might be expected that, as a group, community nurses would be a target for cost savings. In addition, Ackroyd points out that although it would not be accurate to assert that new managers in the NHS took sole responsibility for deciding the content of nurses' work, management decisions had a considerable influence on the amount and kinds of work that nurses were expected to perform.

Outcomes of 'new management' strategies

Whilst accepting Ackroyd's (ibid.) view that the construction of 'new management' systems in the NHS could not be described as Taylorist, that is similar to those first employed by the 'scientific management' movement at the turn of the century in the USA, they have been seen by several commentators (Pollitt 1993, Walby and Greenwell 1994) as a means to control every task involved in the constituent elements of a worker's role. However, as in the main, managers are not nurses, they (the managers) have not possessed the expertise to redesign nursing work. Nevertheless, it is Ackroyd's view that 'new management' has affected the social construction of nursing by circumscribing professional autonomy through the fixing of acceptable levels of cost and budgets. In Ackroyd's opinion, the curtailment of professional autonomy, in respect of community nurses having the authority to determine their own roles in primary health and community care, has eroded their traditional status in the community, caused conflicts between professional attitudes and work experience and created widespread dissatisfaction, a loss of vocationalism, a decrease in recruitment, a loss of morale and a steadily increasing attrition rate (Price Waterhouse 1988, Price Waterhouse et al. 1996).

Symonds and Kelly (1998) also described the effects of organisational change as a result of 'new' management on the work patterns of community nursing. In their view, post-Fordist patterns of work organisation have introduced 'skill mix' models capable of substituting cheaper labour, or less qualified assistants for more qualified staff (NHSME 1992). This is a strategy which seeks to develop a core of highly trained staff with a periphery of less qualified assistants in order to achieve a more flexible workforce. The underlying rationale is that a flexible workforce is essential to respond to the rapidly changing needs encountered in community settings. However, Symonds and Kelly showed that, whilst the resource advantages of this system are obvious, the dangers are that it is likely to undermine the quality of care provided, and compromise the professional responsibilities of nurses. Agreeing with this view, Nettleton (1995:220) also comments that evaluations of skill-mix have found that the overall quality of nursing care is positively related to the qualifications and training of nursing staff and that the quality may be reduced if unqualified staff are overly substituted.

The effects of change on the social construction of community nursing

The above discussions have illustrated how community nurses may have been affected by policy reform and the constraints imposed by other mainly male 'players' such as medical practitioners and managers of health services, a topic that will be returned to later. It would appear that no branch of community nursing has been unscathed by developments, yet each branch may have been affected in a different way, an important consideration in illustrating that the main foci of the various branches of community nursing may be very different in nature. The previous chapter showed how the public health focus of health visiting and school nursing was constrained by the medicalisation of primary care, whilst in this chapter we have seen how the therapeutic caring interventions of district nurses and mental health nurses have also been curtailed by 'managerialism' and the post-Fordist substitution of less qualified workers to provide care. Whilst the demoralising effects of change reported by Ackroyd, and Symonds and Kelly (ibid.) cannnot be denied, Robinson (1992) has shown how community nurses may have attempted to covertly maintain traditional constructs of their roles, and to provide the traditional forms of social care that they have always provided, through supporting the weaker members of society. According to Robinson, managers (and government) are often ignorant of what nurses do, and what they might wish to do, to the extent of regarding nursing as a 'black hole'. As a result, community nurses may still find ways to persist with their traditional ideas of nursing as a profession which is more intent on care than cure, and therefore they are able to find ways of employing their specific expertise to 'enable' rather than 'control' the people who receive their services. In reality, however, Robinson, showed that managerial and medical pressures on nursing practice in community settings may be making the profession increasingly untenable, a possible reason for increasing attrition rates in the profession of community nursing (Clark et al. 2000). One of the reasons given for this speculation is that although care is an integral component of nursing, especially in community settings, little autonomy has been given to community nursing to determine what best constitutes care for the various and sometimes marginalised groups who are the receivers of their services (Kurtz and Wang 1991). As a consequence, community nurses have found themselves being pushed into roles which focus more on cure rather than care and containment and control, rather than roles in which they can provide support for clients who need social nurturance as well as health care intervention, an activity described by Dingwall and Donzelot as a legitimate form of social control (Dingwall et al. 1988). These reflections raise two important questions; the first is, why the professions within community nursing have found it difficult to maintain their philosophical paradigms of practice in the face of medical constructs of primary health care and the pragmatism of managerialism, and the second question is the extent to which their struggles have affected the social construction of their roles.

Traditional conflicts in the construction of nursing roles

In the preface to her book *Gender and the Professional Predicament in Nursing*, Davies (1995) shows how, when nurses speak of the nature of nursing work, their ideals, and of what they need in the way of education and other resources to deliver optimal care, they are often accused of being unrealistic, sentimental, or muddle-headed. Consequently, they have been accused of being 'pretentious' in their borrowings from social science jargon, 'elitist' in their aspirations, and 'defensive' and 'hard to help'. Above all, Davies concludes nurses are 'a frustration and a puzzle to their colleagues in the health field'. She therefore poses the question, of why it is that, although at the point of care delivery nurses are lauded and applauded, collectively in arenas where policy is debated nurses are viewed with ambivalence and negativity? It is Davies' conclusion that this observation can only be due to the fact that the language spoken by nurses has a different root to that of the policy-makers. Because nursing is 'women's work', from a feminist viewpoint it is not difficult to see why the value of community nursing to society is frequently overlooked, undervalued and undermined. These observations may therefore explain why it is that, although community nurses have continued to voice the importance of their preventive and promotive primary health care roles in respect of the implementation of public health strategy and their caring roles in respect of community care provision, the actual formulation of their roles is undoubtedly influenced by medical and managerial constructions, as it is these which strike a concordance with the prevalent male view of government. As Davies observes, despite continual questions related to motivation, morale and recruitment in nursing, and community nursing in particular (Clark et al. 2000), the fundamental discontents of nurses have never been addressed. The confetti of consultation documents and White Papers on future health policy and organisation have, in the main, concerned themselves only with the place of the medical profession in the process of change. Although nurses constitute over half the workforce and their services consume about a quarter of NHS expenditure, nursing has remained marginal to the debates which have shaped health care policy since 1948 (Bearshaw and Robinson 1990:5). For these reasons it is difficult to have confidence in the claims of the profession that they can construct for themselves an active role in the so-called 'second revolution' in health care. Optimism about nursing autonomy to create constructs that fit with their own philosophical paradigms of a caring profession is almost 'strangled at birth' by references to such occurrences as the 1994 RCN annual congress at Brighton reported by Davies (1995). In this vignette, Davies (ibid.) relates how, under the guise of having to save money, speaker after speaker at the conference insisted that highly skilled nurses were not needed for 'shifting paper', giving baths to patients, or holding the hand of a dying person, and of how Christine Hancock, the General Secretary of the College, was a lone voice in arguing that the essence of nursing work was misunderstood, other than by those who may have recently received nursing care and valued the contribution that a highly trained and skilled nurse could make. In Davies' view, therefore, any consideration of how to strengthen the constructions of the role of community nurses in making a valuable contribution to recent developments in health care must take on board that, traditionally, nursing has functioned as an adjunct to the medical profession, enabling it to maintain a masculine-gendered character. As a consequence, the struggles of nursing to become a profession have resulted in nurses emulating achievement of professionalism through the adoption of a masculine-gendered approach. Consequently, this has only served to work against the philosophical constructs of nursing as a caring, rather than a curing profession (albeit one of lesser status than the medical profession). As Gamarnikow (1978:110) pointed out, the role of the nurse, since the turn of the century, has been constructed as one of a helper to the doctor, and relationships between doctor, nurse and patient are repeatedly portrayed as an equation of father/mother/child. Thus, the nurse is constrained to support the doctor rather than the patient in decisions based on what is best for the person needing care. It is the view of Davies, that nursing has been constructed as separate from the knowledge that their work entails, and reconstructed, not as the role of an official of the 'public world', but as an advisor or 'friend' of the family. Thereby, the role of the community nurse as an agent of public control may be conveniently disguised from public view. If, then, community nurses wish to live up to the social construction of their role forwarded by Donzelot (1980), it will surely be necessary for them to portray how it is that they have a capacity to mediate the grievances of social groups constructed as 'excluded' from the nation by virtue of their 'deficiencies'. Also, they need to show how it is that community nursing support can strengthen social discipline and educate the public to deal with the many factors that disrupt health and wellbeing without exerting the more aggressive forms of social control that have been the province of the medical and managerial professions. To date, the experiences of the nursing profession in relation to policy debate over staff recruitment and retention, career progression, education and the organisation of nursing work merely confirm the view that nursing is still seen as an adjunct to the 'real business' of medical care. This construct of the profession makes it difficult for nurses to get to the 'real business' of community nursing care, and to clearly portray the whole spectrum of care that they are capable of providing in order to achieve public health. Blurring of the various roles of community nursing in the guise of increased flexibility will serve only to demean the real value of the rhetoric of collaborative care which currently permeates policy.

Factors influencing the current constructs of community nursing

The 'western model' of health care based on hospitalisation and the importance of medical intervention has been described as an 'engineering model' (McKeown 1976:6). This model is one that creates an analogy of the body as a 'machine' and the health care worker, particularly the doctor, as the scientist or engineer. This model has, for over two centuries, proved its worth especially in crisis interventions and the treatment of acute clinical disorders. However, the complexities of human health and ill health are such that health care and health care services cannot be adequately contained within such a framework. Macdonald (1998) notes how attempts to manage ill health within the framework of westernised models of health care has produced many distortions in the understanding of people's needs. The objectification of disease and ill health has, in Macdonald's opinion, done little to remove suffering caused by psychosocial problems and chronic disease which are major problems in today's society. It is his view that western models of health care are reactive rather than proactive, that there is an emphasis on waiting for something to go wrong, a sense of waiting to pickup the broken pieces, rather than to provide pre-emptive care. In fact, westernised medicine has also been described by Macdonald as a 'fire-brigade' approach whereby most of the scarce resources for health care and social interventions are spent on hospital treatment which is costly and increasingly inaccessible to many in the population. This 'westernised' model of health care intervention has been increasingly criticised for its inability to create health, and its focus on individual biology and physiology rather than the socio-economic context in which the individual has to operate. Recent research in social medicine (Benzeval et al. 1995) continues to show that health improves as people get wealthier, therefore investment in community resources may be more appropriate than technological care. As Acheson (DoH 1998b:1) noted, current health problems are primarily a matter of social justice. Although the past twenty years have brought a marked increase in prosperity and substantial reductions in mortality to the people of this country as a whole, the gap in health between those at the top and bottom of the social scale has widened.

The NHS and Community Care Act of 1990 appeared to be the culmination of decades of dissatisfaction with westernised models of health care, and for many it provided tangible proof of a shift away from the medical professions' hegemonic control of defining and controlling health. The Act was welcomed as a desirable objective for service users and providers (Means and Smith 1994). The White paper *Caring for People* (DoH 1989a:9) stated that:

> Community care means providing the right level of intervention and support to enable people to achieve maximum independence and control over their own lives....For this aim to become a reality, the development of a wide range of services provided in a variety of settings is essential. These services form part of a spectrum of care ranging from domiciliary support provided to people in their own homes to residential and nursing homes and long stay hospital care for those for whom other forms of care are no longer enough.

Similarly the Act promised many changes in health care which were additional to the significant move away from institutional care. Specifically, the re-emergence of an emphasis on the public health role within the World Health Organisation's broad vision of primary health care including environmental change, preventive care, personal services and health education, signalled public health and primary care partnerships which would require major changes in practice over and above the simple accommodation of public health.

Successive legislation throughout the 1990s has gradually reinforced the shift away from institutional care, and western medicine's hegemonic insistence on the value of cure rather than care. Reference to Foucault's thesis 'regimes of truth' (Foucault 1980, see Chapter 1) shows that the shift away from westernised medicine is not such a startling occurrence as those of us brought up in the scientific era might wish to believe. It is his contention that every society at specific historical periods produces an all-enveloping 'truth' to which people will adhere. This 'truth' is a product of people's reality and it is transmitted through a variety of discourses, such has been the discourse of 'westernised medicine'. However, whereas in the twentieth century the human body became the site of medical and scientific practice justifying a powerful control on, and over, the individual human body and its function, sometimes described as the 'clinical gaze', in the twenty-first century a new 'truth' is emerging. This 'truth' appears to convey that health and wellbeing are dependent on the control of 'social spaces' (Armstrong 1995), that is, it is the social determinants of health which need to be tackled (Figure 5.1) if health status is to improve. As Acheson (DoH 1998b) has shown 'the root causes of

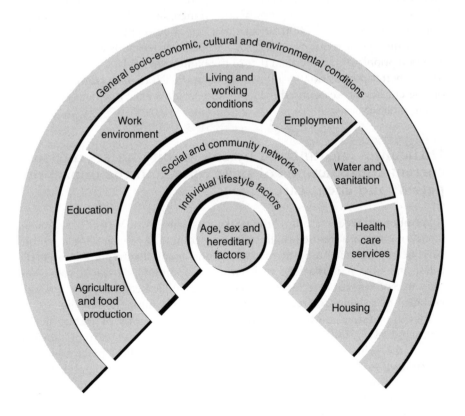

Figure 5.1 The main determinants of health

Source: Dahlgren, G. (1996)

health' must be tackled if health is to improve. It is his contention that this can only be done by adopting a socio-economic model of health care, as scientific evidence shows that health inequalities are the outcome of causal chains which run back into and from the basic structure of society. Health care policies should therefore be both 'upstream' and 'downstream':

> For instance, a policy which reduces inequalities in income and improves the income of the less well off, and one which provides pre-school education for all four year olds are examples of 'upstream' policies which are likely to have a wide range of consequences, including benefits to health. Policies such as providing nicotine replacement therapy on prescription, or making available better facilities for taking physical exercise, are 'downstream' interventions which have a narrower range of benefits. (DoH 1998b)

Both 'upstream' and 'downstream' policies which deal with wider influences on health inequalities such as income distribution, education, public safety, housing, work environments, employment, social networks, transport and pollution, as well as those which have narrower impacts, such as healthy behaviours, have, in Acheson's opinion, the capacity to reduce death rates considerably. Certainly such policies have greater potential to improve health status than the reduction of 'waiting times' and an increase in the number of operations performed (DoH 2000). Social care has the potential to reduce death rates in the lowest social class, and since this currently stands at 50 deaths per 100,000 population, more than that of the highest social class, it would appear to be a better proposition to adopt such an approach than to continue to rely on the efficacy of westernised medicine to provide a cure for society's lack of caring interventions.

Difficulties encountered by community nurses due to current constructions of their roles, and the impact on patient and client care

A number of recent studies undertaken as part of a Master's degree in Collaborative Care are used to illustrate how community nursing interventions have been restricted by both managerial and medical interpretations of the roles, and how it is that the real nature of community nursing roles, and the value of nursing care interventions to the public health may be seriously curtailed by a failure to create a true construct of community nursing.

In a qualitative study of health visitors' perceptions of public health practice, Lewis (2000), showed how health visiting practice, currently located within the primary care team and dominated by medical practitioners, is constrained from achieving collective community approaches to public health, and from provision of a model of care directed at the level of the individual or family rather than the community at large. It was Lewis' view that the main constraints imposed on health visitors were a lack of time for involvement in public health activity due to the pressures and demands of an unyielding caseload (often determined by managerial and medical constructs of the health visiting role) (Symonds and Kelly 1998) and the undemocratic power relationships within the PHC team which undermine effective team working and the adoption of a collaborative, community-focused approach to care. It was also discovered that, far from being confident about their particular construct of health visiting, health visitors proposed different interpretations of what was required of a 'public health' role and 'public health' practice were identified. Lewis therefore concluded that many of the health visitors who took part in her study felt inadequately prepared for their role and lacked the skills and expertise to undertake, in a confident manner, collective approaches to public health care. In order to equip health visitors with a more definite construction of their role so that they could provide an autonomous response to the demands of current policy, it was recommended by Lewis that:

a common understanding of the concept and process of public health is developed, so that 'interested others' will understand health visitors' interpretations of their role;

an 'ideal model' of public health is articulated through resolution of the different features of selective models of PHC favoured by many in the medical and administrative professions and the comprehensive models of PHC favoured by the social interpretevists;

the education of health visitors is firmly focused on the development of public health practice;

there is a need to raise awareness at a strategic level that perfunctory concessions to public health practice are insufficient to improve health care, and that planned, well managed and re-educative change is required if health visitors are to be enabled to present an amalgam of 'unseen, private needs' which call for public health interventions, thereby empowering and enabling disadvantaged groups rather than controlling them;

there is a need for an examination and exploration of new ways of working if the effectiveness of a combined generic and public health role for health visitors is to be maintained;

the morale of the profession needs to be raised in the light of the above recommendations and that this should be achieved through a review of health visitor education, and supported professional development;

clearer role definitions should reflect current policy and adopt a community development role.

These findings clearly reflect the observations of Davies (1995) and confirm that subjective role insecurity on the part of health visitors is undoubtedly an outcome of the constraints placed upon the profession by other more powerful groups. As a consequence, it is suggested that the perceived ability of health visitors to provide the community with supportive interventions which engender social discipline maybe seriously hampered by the fact that they are being coerced into the provision of an intrusive rather than an enabling form of social control in order to achieve the goals of a masculine-dominated service.

In a study of the boundaries between health and social care which have emerged since the NHS and Community Care Act (1990), A.M. Jones (2000) examined the problems experienced by district nurses providing care for patients with Multiple Sclerosis, a chronic degenerative disease. It was clearly shown in this study that boundaries constructed between the provision of health and social care, and the mistaken belief that highly qualified nurses should not be involved in the 'menial' tasks of caring, have resulted in fragmentation in the provision of care, and the loss of the individual as the main focus of care. Commodification of care provision through the construction of packages of care was shown to have resulted in gaps in provision, on the one hand, and duplication of services on the other. In addition, the fracture of the continuous relationship between health and social care provision has led to plenty of opportunities for 'passing the buck' between health and social care providers and communication problems and difficulties in the coordination of care. It was concluded that the increasing complexities experienced by district nurses caring for patients in community settings require alternative solutions to those currently available. Recommendations for change were that more consideration needs to be given to the interpretation of the meaning of health, and health determinants. The causes of gaps and duplication in services need to be identified and remedied, caring interventions need to be refocused on the needs of the patients rather than the services, and knowledge and skills need to be shared so that continuity of care is achieved. In addition, Jones recommends that information flow between the various services is streamlined, and the complexities of providing a flexible and responsive service explored. Access to services should be simplified and the need for a gate keeper role in the light of multiple providers and pluralism in care investigated. Risk sharing, trust and commitment have to be defined and explored and, finally, the increasing role of carers has to be considered and facilitated in an empowering way. Thus, this study shows how constraints on the role of the district nurse are also affecting standards of community care. It also demonstrates the specific differences in the foci of health visiting and district nursing roles, thereby indicating that the desire to increase the flexibility of community nursing through the blurring of roles and shared educational programmes can only lead to inferior standards of care, and a possible decline of public confidence in the nursing profession.

In another study of district nursing S. Jones (2000), showed how a departure of community nurses from a caring role was undermining public support. Specifically the incidence of verbal abuse experienced by this branch of community nursing has increased as a consequence of restrictions imposed on the provision of services. A survey of 50 district nurses showed that over a period of six months these nurses had experienced a total of 206 incidents of verbal abuse from patients. Some 34 of these incidents had not been reported to anyone whereas of the other 172 incidents 11 per cent had been verbally reported to the employer, 47 per cent to a team leader, and 42 per cent to another nurse; none of the incidents were formally documented. It was also shown that most abuse is directed at the most senior nurses in the team and is instigated by men who are usually of the same age as the nurse. Usually the abuse takes place in the patient's home. It is concluded that, as a result of the implementation of the NHS and Community Care Act (1990), the Patients Charter (1991) and Carer's Act (2001), unrealistic expectations may have been constructed of district nurses and of the resources and services that they are now able to provide. As a consequence of being seen as 'the face of the health service' and perceived as the barrier to receipt of what patients define as their rights, district nurses receive verbal abuse. Recommending that community nurses are trained to deal with this form of aggression and that Trusts and Health Authorities should produce guidelines to protect staff, improve management strategies and provide post-incident support, this study misses the point that violence may be the result of the constraints placed on the autonomy of the district nurse, and the subjugation of a caring role which engenders social responsibility to a role that is more concerned with control and management of aggression caused by dissatisfaction with resources, rather than nursing interventions.

Finally, in a paper on the social deconstruction of community learning disability nursing (CLD), Sumner and Sumner (2000) show that, as a result of constraints on resource provision, CLD teams have begun to fragment and lose their focus. These writers contend that failure to review and reorientate the role of CLD nurses to the needs of community care policy has resulted in role subjugation by commissioners and care managers which has implications in terms of the security and clarity of the future role of this group of nurses.

It is concluded from all of the above examples that the current constructions of the roles of community nurses have been seriously impaired by the actions of others, and that the focus on caring has been subjugated to the need for a flexible workforce whose purpose is to support medical and managerial goals rather than care for people's health and social needs.

Role re-alignment

To overcome the problems outlined above and to realistically engage in a second revolution in community nursing as was suggested in Chapter 2, community nurses need to articulate the true meanings of the concepts of health and primary health care (Macdonald 1992), and the extent to which increasing social inequalities are seriously affecting the nation's health (Popay et al. in Bartley et al. 1998). Symmonds and Kelly (1998) showed how imperative it is for community nurses to re-enter the world of public health and social care and strengthen their image as community workers (see Chapter 3). Clarke, in Symmonds and Kelly (1998) suggests that the way forward for community nurses, in terms of reconstructing their roles and overcoming the oppression of governmentality is to involve themselves in the process of community development for health. It is Clarke's contention that community development presents an opportunity for community nurses to play a full part in the organisation and management of new forms of social care in the community, in partnership and as experts rather than as dispensers of elixirs. This suggests that the role requirements of community nurses should be the ability to provide social care and support in its many and various forms of intervention as well as, or instead of, participating in curing interventions. On a positive note, it is reassuring to see that community nurses have already recognised the challenges of community development approaches to care, and the important contributions that these can make to society. Such approaches are discussed in detail in Chapter 6.

Conclusion

This chapter has argued that the efforts of community nurses to construct an image of themselves as an empowering profession have been seriously hampered by their own readiness to conform with the perceptions of others. Specifically, government strategy, managerial pragmatism, the influence of the medical profession and issues of gendered identity have been examined and shown to be important drawbacks to the autonomy of community nurses to portray themselves as public carers. Several studies have been employed to illustrate this point, and it is concluded that the image that has been constructed as the result of these constraints may have done much to confirm that community nurses are more concerned with the maintenance of social order amongst those groups in society which are excluded from full participation in social life, than they are with the inclusion of these groups into mainstream public involvement, through processes of caring social control. It has been suggested that a means of reconstructing the roles of community nursing would be by grasping the challenge of public health and community development, particularly for the socially excluded sectors of society. The following chapter examines the extent to which community nurses are rising to this challenge.

CHAPTER 6

The Front-Line: Community Nursing, Policies of Community and Governmentality

Introduction

This chapter is concerned with three main issues: the current direction and meaning of policies which place the restoration of community and social inclusion at their centre; the vulnerable groups at whom these policies are directed; and the real lived experience of community nurses and health visitors who, as ever, are placed in the front-line of the administration of social order. Since the elections of the New Labour administrations in 1997 and 2001, policies have shown a continuation of former emphases on efficiency, value for money and economy but this has been coupled with a desire to tackle the causes of social exclusion. There has been in many respects a revival of public health, with the first appointment of a Minister of Public Health. This higher profile was carried in individual policy documents on the state of the nation's health in England, Wales and Scotland. Interestingly, in all the documents the structural causes of ill health such as poverty, bad housing, unemployment, low income and lack of educational opportunities were focused upon as well as a recognition that personal circumstances and culture had an effect on lifestyles. This was a break with the almost sole fixation on personal risk and a 'blaming the victim' attitude which was prevalent in the *The Health of the Nation* (DoH 1992) document. But, as we shall see, the new direction of policies presents a puzzle for management and community practitioners, it requires a shift of focus and a corresponding cultural change.

Many of the new policies, which address the problem of social exclusion, present an enhanced role for community-based nursing and health visiting. However, as we shall see, the division between social and health care within the branches of community nursing has become more clearly defined. The targeting of groups who are vulnerable to social exclusion such as problem families and teenage mothers, as well as the provision of long-term care for elderly people, those with severe mental health problems, and the chronic sick, have placed all branches of community nursing in the forefront of the implementation of policies.

145

How do those who are in the front-line in the provision of care and the implementation of policies of preventing and tackling social exclusion experience this new responsibility? Drawing from a selection of research studies of the daily experiences of those providing care and implementing new services, the voices of those in the front-line will be heard.

Health inequalities – causes and solutions

Social inequality and its impact on collective and individual health has been the basis of the creation and development of public health in Britain for over a century. Ill health, high infant mortality, prevalence of disease and early death have always been connected to poverty and deprivation. The welfare state and, specifically, the National Health Service were conceived as the solution to this seemingly inevitable situation. The postwar economic boom and increasing affluence especially among the working classes and the less well off, coupled with the universal access to health care, education, housing and welfare appeared for a short period to have addressed the legacy of poverty and ill health. The publication of the Black Report in 1980 (DoH 1980a) once more pinpointed wide variations in health between the social classes and between regions. Various studies throughout the 1980s and 1990s (Moylan et al. 1984, Townsend et al. 1992, Wilkinson 1997) evidenced the 'health gap' between income groups. The response of successive administrations throughout this time was to focus upon *individual* causes for the widespread inequalities. Lifestyle theories abounded and people were, in a sense, 'blamed' for their own ill health. Diet, smoking, excessive alcohol consumption and lack of exercise ranked high in the 'causes' of premature deaths from cancer and heart disease. However, the *structural* causes; poverty, unemployment, bad housing, industrial pollution, were hardly, if ever, mentioned in health promotion leaflets which exhorted people to 'Look After Yourself'. This approach was criticised by writers such as Ashton and Seymour (1988) who argued for a 'new' public health which would take account of structural causes which individuals were powerless to combat. This approach involved health visitors, health promotion advisors, and other community health workers to move beyond the targeting of individual behaviour and to engage in wider campaigns for the improvement of neighbourhood facilities and conditions. But the overall drive and direction of policies to 'improve' health remained at the individual level and the organisational structure of community nursing and health visiting during this time was firmly based upon the achievement of individual 'targets' and narrowly focused upon individual caseloads. Widespread inequalities of health therefore became defined as the result of the ignorance, perversity or sheer unwillingness of the poor to 'help themselves'. Nowhere was this more illustrated than in *The Health of the Nation* (DoH 1992) which became the blueprint for managerial systems of implementation of this narrow concentration upon individual 'healthy or risky behaviour' and the negation of structural issues such as poverty.

This direction and definition changed with the publication, in 1998, of the three UK White Papers on the state of the nation's health. The Papers which, following devolution, separately addressed England in *Our Healthier Nation* (DoH 1998a), Wales (Better Health – Better Wales) (WO. 1998) and Scotland (*Working Together for a Healthier Scotland*) (SO. 1998), all contained the universal message that poverty was the single largest cause of ill health. Once the *cause* of wide spread inequalities had been defined as structural rather than merely individual then the *solutions* were also correspondingly more varied and of a radically different nature. All three Papers focused upon the long-term health effects of childhood poverty and of locality-based deprivation which affected the health of whole communities who shared the characteristics of poverty and hopelessness. What was of the greatest concern was the fact that, despite an overall growth in living standards throughout the previous 20 years, health inequalities and poverty rates had actually increased since 1979. In the late 1970s, less than one in ten of the population lived below the EC poverty line (calculated as less than half average income) but by the late 1990s, this had risen to one in four. The problem was not evenly spread, poverty rates being highest in the post-industrial areas of Wales, Scotland and the North East of England as well as some areas of London. But it was amongst children that poverty rates were the highest. Government statistics showed that a third of Britain's children are born into poverty (DSS 1998). All other factors associated with childhood deprivation and ill health follow from this disadvantage. The cycle of poverty and disadvantage is strong and even extends to conditions pre-birth, malnutrition in pregnancy affects later adult susceptibility to chronic diseases such as heart disease, stroke and chronic chest diseases. Research has shown that inequalities at each early stage in life affect adult health rates (Power et al. 1991).

In 1997, the incoming New Labour government commissioned a new review of evidence of health inequalities and proposals for strategies to combat the causes of widespread deprivation. Published in late 1998, the Acheson Report (DoH 1998b), adopted a 'socio-economic model' of health, which placed individuals at the centre of circles of influential factors which all determine health. These other layers of influence include the surrounding community cultures, living and working conditions, access to goods and services, food standards, and wider economic and environmental conditions. Whilst the individual is 'endowed with age, sex and constitutional factors which undoubtedly influence their health potential, but which are fixed' (DoH 1998b:3), the surrounding layers 'could be modified'. Based upon this definition of causes of health inequalities, the Acheson Report recommended a wide range of policies and programmes which illustrated the need to intervene on a broad front to address the problem. This intervention included; the increase in benefits, especially income support to tackle child poverty, improvement in social housing standards and accessibility, tackling of street crime, improvement of public transport and reduction of car usage, reduction of food and fuel poverty especially among the elderly, and extension of pre-school education to poorer families and the provision of quality childcare and the improvement of employment opportunities and working conditions. This proposed interventionist programme cut across traditional departmental boundaries of health, social security, education and employment, housing and environment and the Home Office. Social policies were to be 'joined up'. This wide front included new Welfare to Work programmes for young people, changes to payments to working families from Family Credit to the Working Families Tax Credit, the introduction of a minimum wage, childcare payments to single mothers who took employment, and the introduction of a Food Agency in 1999 to monitor food standards.

In 2002, the Government continued with this approach setting up a consultation exercise aimed at *Tackling Health Inequalities* (DoH 2002a). The NHS Plan in 2000 had set targets for national health inequalities on areas such as reducing smoking, reducing teenage conceptions, and tackling child poverty. The approach was to tackle disadvantage on a community-wide scale. In responses to the exercise, the necessity for community development was strongly articulated.

But the task of intervention within communities and with families to attempt to halt the continuation of disadvantage lies with the health service, local Trusts and Health Authorities, the voluntary sector and social services. Within the sphere of the health service an 'enhanced' role for community practitioners, especially health visitors and school nurses, is explicitly set out.

Community regeneration

As we saw in Chapter 3, the construction of communities in terms of locality and housing was achieved through social policies. But as these *ascribed* communities were structured by the local economy and were organised around the centrality of the male breadwinner, so the decline of heavy industries and the fragmentation of the model family and cohesive neighbourhoods followed from economic change in the 1980s. Many of the communities within which community nurses practise contain only remnants of the respectable working-class areas of the 1950s. In some areas, the only people who have had experience of work are now in their sixties and are often the grandparents (or more usually great-grandparents) to families who are workless. Many grandmothers in these deprived areas are providing the only resource of childcare and support for isolated and unsupported mothers. Anyone accompanying a health visitor to these areas will witness at first hand the sense of isolation and hopelessness that pervades family life. Teenage motherhood has become a 'norm', with the prospect of becoming a grandmother the only ambition of women who are in their late twenties (Hunt 2001, Symonds 2003). Poverty, deprivation, unemployment and social exclusion are now third generational. In addition to these post-industrial areas there are many inner-city estates that have become virtual 'no-go' areas, 'dangerous places' where young men roam in packs and lawlessness is a way of life. The publicised murder of ten year old Damilola Taylor in South London in 2001 vividly illustrated the continued existence of the 'problem area'.

This situation requires government action on a wide scale. There is no one solution but a multi-agency and cross-cutting approach is essential. These are areas of social exclusion that lack a community culture of participation and active citizenship. It is here that a wide-ranging approach covering health inequalities, education and training needs, employment opportunities, poor housing, crime reduction and environmental renewal is needed. The Social Exclusion Unit (2000) published its strategy for neighbourhood renewal based on preventing social exclusion and involving a high level of community participation (DETR 1997). The main drive behind all policies is the belief in paid work as the solution to on-going poverty. The drive to construct a skilled, educated and flexible workforce underpins all connected policies and strategies, especially that of Sure Start. The ability to work is now defined as a basis for active citizenship and a value to be transmitted by responsible parents. This represents a sea-change in assumptions upon which the welfare state was based, the male breadwinner and the supported and dependent wife whose role was to provide unpaid care for the family.

The characteristics of citizenship and the new policy direction aimed at promoting citizenship in regenerated communities can be seen in Figure 6.1.

New discourses and new welfare

In her address to the annual conference of the CPHVA in 1998, Professor Ruth Lister set out the main components of the government's approach to welfare reform and a 'rethinking of the welfare state'. In this address, she pinpointed the main themes underlying policy as; equality of opportunity rather than greater equality as such, responsibilities over rights as part of a new contract for welfare, paid work as the primary means to social inclusion, joined-up policy-making, as exemplified by the work of the Social Exclusion Unit and the shifting of resources from cash benefits to services (Lister 1999:19).

As well as these themes that undoubtedly run through the direction of policies, there are also discernible discourses which can be said to overarch and permeate both the meaning and implementation of policies. We would identify the dominant discourses as;

- social exclusion and inclusion,
- work,
- responsible families,
- modernisation.

All of these have significance for the work and 'enhanced role' of community nurses and health visitors in the implementation of policies. In the previous

Figure 6.1 Characteristics of citizenship and new policy directions

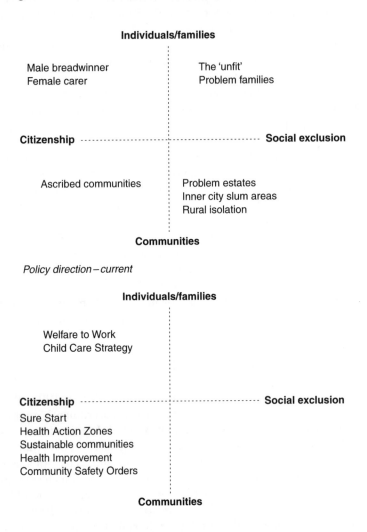

Individuals/families

Male breadwinner
Female carer

The 'unfit'
Problem families

Citizenship ---------------------------- Social exclusion

Ascribed communities

Problem estates
Inner city slum areas
Rural isolation

Communities

Policy direction – current

Individuals/families

Welfare to Work
Child Care Strategy

Citizenship ---------------------------- Social exclusion

Sure Start
Health Action Zones
Sustainable communities
Health Improvement
Community Safety Orders

Communities

chapter we looked at the significance of definitions of social exclusion and at the culture of localities and groups that have become marginalised. The significance of this discourse for present policies is the addition of the concept of the *predictability* of future exclusion. Studies such as the National Child Development Study by Hobcraft (1998) shows in detail the links between childhood circumstances and indicators of social exclusion. In summary, this analysis shows the four most consistent childhood factors as being;

● childhood poverty,
● family disruption,

- evidence of contact with the police,
- low educational test score.

In addition, the chances of an adult life lived on benefit are increased by;

- poor performance at school and lack of parental interest – especially fathers' interest in boys,
- disrupted family circumstances – especially for girls, any experience of being taken into care.

The increased chance of teenage pregnancy, is, of course, heavily related to the above factors. Recent data on school exclusions reveal a similar pattern, with boys in the vast majority of those excluded. The concept of 'modern malnutrition' has been used to describe the situation in areas of social exclusion which have been defined as 'food deserts', with, in some instances, drugs being more easily attainable than fresh fruit or vegetables (Leather 1996, DoH 1998b). Clearly there is a great and enhanced role for health visitors and other practitioners in the tackling of these problems which are detailed in policies. The discourse of social exclusion is linked to its solution – social inclusion. But how to bring the excluded in from the cold? The present government has signalled that there is only one long-term solution – work.

The discourse of the value of work in both an economic and a moral sense permeates policies. Unlike the Beveridge Plan that set the foundations for the postwar welfare state, the value of work and the necessity of wage earning is no longer confined to men. The construction of the 'male breadwinner' model of welfare and the labour market that dominated British life has been replaced by the model of the 'universal worker'. The identity of a 'dependent' has been withdrawn from women, including those with school-age children and extended to single mothers with pre-school children. Partners of unemployed males and single mothers are included in the Welfare to Work regulations, and the reduction of the single-parent allowance plus the funding of a system of public childcare, all signal a great cultural change.

> Worklessness is the most common cause of poverty among working age people and their children. Moving into employment is the surest route out of poverty. (Treasury 2000)

But for many in the deprived and post-industrial areas, this is not an easy cultural change to adopt. The ideology of the male breadwinner remains stubbornly strong even though the economic base for this belief no longer exists. In many of the post-industrial areas of South Wales, for example, there are proportionally more women than men currently in the workforce even though most work in low-paid and unskilled occupations. In many areas there is now a 'feminised' labour market which means that many jobs previously thought of as 'women's work' are now being sought by unemployed men.

There is clearly a role for health visiting, school nursing, community psychiatric nurses and others in supporting families in undertaking work, in the encouragement of young people and women to undertake training and education and in the support and counselling of young men in the controlling of violence and depression. The third discourse is inextricably linked to those of social exclusion and work.

There is evidence from government policies that a redefinition of the 'responsible family' is also being constructed. Although an emphasis on the married nuclear family structure as the 'preferred option' within which to bring up children remains, nevertheless, a more tolerant and open approach to other partnerships and sexual relationships is evidenced. The reduction in the age of consent for male homosexuality, the parity given to unmarried partners in cases of domestic violence, all point to a more open attitude. But this is counterbalanced by a much publicised concern over teenage pregnancy. Although a specific Ministry of the Family has not been created, family policies are a prominent part of policy-making. Previously hidden issues such as domestic violence and childcare have been given a high profile and specifically delegated to health professionals in *Supporting Families* (Home Office 1998). Parental responsibility is the focus of widespread legislation including curfew orders on children under 10, parental prosecution for persistent truancy, school–parent contracts over homework, and the Criminal Justice Act of 1998 which made parental responsibility for the debts of children under 18 a legal requirement. But it is the relatively high incidence of teenage pregnancy that is the focus of governmental concern. It is evident from research that the risk factors for teenage pregnancy are discernible, and are linked to all other factors of social exclusion.

The concept of 'modernisation' is one which has been used frequently both in the titles of government documents such as *Modernising Mental Health Services* (DoH 1999) and in publicised speeches by the Prime Minister,

> We believe in active government and we believe in public service, but if government is going to be effective at delivering services in the way people want them today, it has to be modernised, it has to be updated. (Cabinet Office 1999)

This discourse of modernisation is essentially one of organisation. It is the management and organisational structure of the public services which is to be 'modernised'. What does this actually mean for the delivery of community services? We look at this point in depth in the second part of this book but we would argue that its meaning includes a change in both the practice and culture of both managers and community practitioners. One element of this new way of working is the rejection of the traditional profession-led approach and the top-down style of decision-making. The relationship between users of a service and the professional is to change and become a more participatory one. The breaking down of inter-professional barriers has become a reality for many working in the field of community care and child protection, and this is now set to continue into many of the new community-based programmes. Before we go on to look in detail at some of these programmes which are being targeted at specific groups, it is necessary to first set out a model of policies which illustrate this new direction.

Models and direction of policies

The direction of policies implemented since 1998 have shown a significant shift towards a community-based approach and away from a focus upon the individual. This shift is of great significance to the organisational and management structure of community services as well as signalling a cultural change. As demonstrated in Figure 6.2, the importance of this shift can be appreciated when a comparison is drawn between policies from the early 1990s to the present.

There are some caveats to make however when analysing this general trend towards community- and client-based services; the overwhelming funding and focus within the health service remains with hospital services and there is a clear division opening up between what could be termed *social intervention* and *health care provision*. The overwhelming policy shift towards social inclusion has meant that health visitors, school nurses and, to an extent, community pyschiatric nurses, have become involved in what is primarily social intervention, support and control with socially vulnerable groups, whilst the

Figure 6.2 Public health policies, 1992–2000

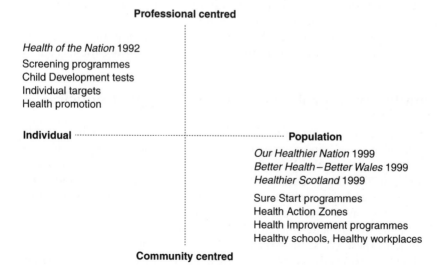

Professional centred

Health of the Nation 1992
Screening programmes
Child Development tests
Individual targets
Health promotion

Individual   **Population**

Our Healthier Nation 1999
Better Health – Better Wales 1999
Healthier Scotland 1999

Sure Start programmes
Health Action Zones
Health Improvement programmes
Healthy schools, Healthy workplaces

Community centred

Figure 6.3 Social support and nursing provision

Community-based support/intervention	Individual-based care/nursing
Providers	
Health visitors	District nurses
School nurses	Nursing care support staff
	Community psychiatric nurses
Targeted groups	
Vulnerable families	Long-term care for elderly and the
Teenage mothers	mentally ill and severely disabled.
	Short-term care for post-operative cases,
Aims	
Social inclusion – eradication of	Care in community – alternative to
future social inequality and poverty	institutional and hospital provision

district nursing and nursing support services are firmly placed in the provision of health and nursing care to others. This pattern is illustrated in Figure 6.3.

As can be seen, the dominant trend within health policies is towards a population/community-centred approach (Figure 6.2), but within community nursing itself there is a further division between the 'public' nature of social interventionist policies aimed at 'social problems' and the 'private' nature of individually- and home-based nursing care for people in need (Figure 6.3). Community nursing is being clearly separated by policy aims into two different and discrete segments. This is at a time when inter-professional collaboration is being encouraged and extended and the pooling of social service and health budgets are taking place within local authorities. The picture is therefore complex and appears at times to be contradictory.

We turn now to look in detail at the new roles for community nurses within these policies and at how nurses themselves are experiencing these changes.

Families with problems – the new support policies

Publicised concerns over the future of 'the family' and predictions of its decline formed an important part of political rhetoric throughout the 1980s and 1990s. During the New Right administrations the rhetoric tended to focus upon a 'return to traditional family values' and the stigmatisation of single mothers as being welfare dependent, feckless and irresponsible (Murray 1994). This was of course the basis of the attack by Murray on the construction by the welfare state and feminist ideas of the 'underclass'. But despite the rhetoric of these years, the restructuring of the 'traditional' family had been an ongoing process throughout the postwar years. In 1961, the proportion of 'traditional' households in Britain (a married couple with dependent children) was 38 per cent but by 1998, this had fallen to only 25 per cent. By the end of the century, childless couples outnumbered those with dependent children and the number of single person households had risen to nearly 30 per cent. The number of 'traditional' families of dependent children, with two adults, one of whom is in work, has fallen by a third since 1981 (Rowntree Foundation 1995).

But the decline of marriage and the increase in divorce coupled with the overall fall in the birth rate only served to focus upon those families who were headed by a lone parent, usually the mother (by 1995 there were half the number of marriages and twice the number of divorces than in 1975). By 1998, the proportion of lone-parent families was around 22 per cent, representing 1.7 million families with approaching 3 million children (Social Trends 1998). The highest number of lone mothers are divorced or separated (57 per cent) with 38 per cent being never married. But of course marriage is not the only indicator of 'unsupported' motherhood, the highest percentage of babies born to unmarried parents are, nevertheless, jointly registered with only 18 per cent of never-married mothers having never lived with their partner (Joseph Rowntree Foundation 1997). But it is the connection between children and family poverty that has become the focus of policies. Since 1981, the number of families with two adults, neither of whom are in work, has risen by 25 per cent. This represents a polarisation in British society between what has become called the 'work rich/work poor' divide. One child in ten in Britain (over one million) lives in a household where no adult is in receipt of a wage. Furthermore, these 'work poor' families are also concentrated into specific localities in social housing, where this situation is the 'norm'. This must be contrasted to other localities where it is unique to find any child living in a wageless family. The division between families in work is also complex. As Hilary Land has shown, although poverty is concentrated in lone-mother families, it is also to be found in two-parent families in work. One third of the families dependent upon income support in 1997 were headed by a man, and in nearly half of all families claiming Family Credit in 1998, the main earner was a man (Land 1999:129). The disappearance of full-time jobs for the male manual working class has been of enormous financial and cultural significance. The 'demise of the male breadwinner and the rise of the lone mother' (Land 1999:129) represents the greatest upheaval and challenge to the postwar welfare state.

The perceived problem of family and child poverty, its visibility, causation and perpetuation lies at the heart of new policies. In 1999, the Prime Minister, Tony Blair announced,

> Our historic aim will be that ours will be the first generation to end child poverty... it is a twenty year mission. (Quoted in Piachaud 1999)

The government approach is two fold; to engage upon a programme of income distribution through fiscal measures, and to intervene to support families in parenting, childcare and tackling domestic violence – in other words to *socialise* people into the values of work and responsible citizenship.

The twin discourses of work and responsibility are constantly evoked in the fiscal and social measures which are being undertaken to address poverty and its corollary – social exclusion. The Working Families Tax Credit, additional child-care credit, the Welfare to Work programme and the national childcare strategy are the three of the proposed key routes out of poverty and into social inclusion. But coupled with these redistributive measures targeted at the poorest, there is also a programme of intervention and support for 'families' in general.

As the Home Secretary, Jack Straw, stated in his Foreword to the consultative document *Supporting Families*,

> But what families – all families – have a right to expect from government is support. (Home Office 1999)

In Figure 6.4, we can illustrate this new direction by the use of the model employed in Figure 6.2. Within this new approach, we can see that the role of health visitors is central. Indeed, this 'enhanced and expanding' role is flagged up at the beginning of the document. The nature of this expanded role is also clearly set out: 'The expanded role of health visitors would involve a shift of emphasis from *dealing with* problems to *preventing* problems arising in the first place.'

As the document itself noted, many health visitors are already engaged in providing a range of advice on matters, but now they are required to be

Figure 6.4   New approaches towards working with vulnerable families

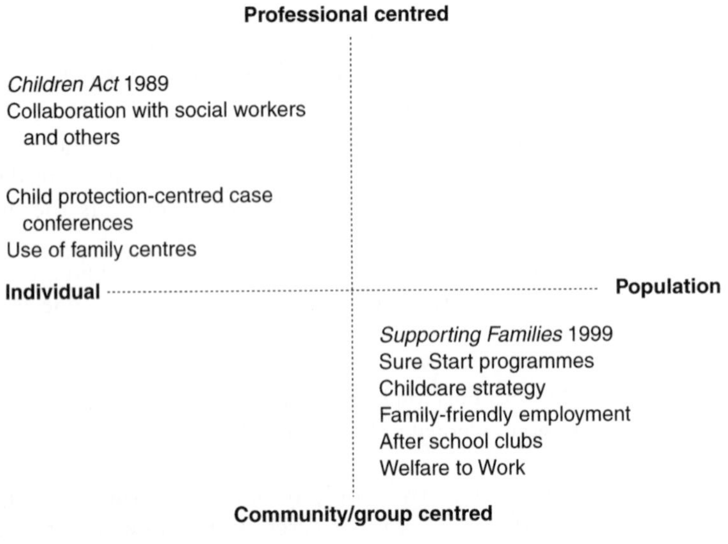

Professional centred

Children Act 1989
Collaboration with social workers
   and others

Child protection-centred case
   conferences
Use of family centres

Individual ··· **Population**

Supporting Families 1999
Sure Start programmes
Childcare strategy
Family-friendly employment
After school clubs
Welfare to Work

Community/group centred

involved with community-based programmes which are state funded and evaluated. This is, we believe, a new direction for health visiting. The emphasis is away from its more recent site of the home-based visit focused upon a narrow definition of 'health' and into a wider remit of social support akin in many ways to that of its original practice of the late nineteenth century. The 'problems' mentioned in the Green Paper are not specifically those of 'health' but more concerned with the acquisition of social skills and civic responsibility.

The Sure Start programme, which is targeted at areas of greatest need, requires health visitors to work in conjunction with many other agencies and workers. This, in itself, is a break from the traditional 'universalism' of the service. Sure Start is specifically aimed at families who are experiencing or who live in areas of perceived and connected social problems. It is a wide-ranging programme which is aimed to support parents in many ways such as: training for work, help with literacy and numeracy, help with parenting problems, with postnatal depression and other emotional difficulties. As Hilary Graham has argued:

> The Sure Start programme is one example of an intervention designed to lift children in disadvantaged circumstances onto more advantaged trajectories. However, as a targeted rather than universal intervention, it will only reach around 5% of children aged three years and under. (Graham 1999:14)

In her address to the CPHVA conference, Graham recognised that despite the move to targeted provision a universal service is also required. The role of management in this shift towards community-based programmes of support and the role of health visitors remains crucial. The inability or unwillingness of management to move from the 'old' ways of working to the new approach is one which is, in some areas, excluding health visitors from involvement in the Sure Start programme. Of the first wave of 21 Sure Start programmes begun in 1999, only two were health authority led. This has led to worries about health visitor exclusion from the programmes in many areas due to management reluctance to participate (Community Practitioner 1999:111). The organisational shift required is one of a change of culture in management and practitioners. Later in this chapter, the experiences of a group of health visitors engaged in attempting to change the traditional approach will be described.

The concern over disadvantaged families cannot, of course, be divorced from one of the overriding moral panics of the 1980s and 1990s, the issue of teenage pregnancy.

Teenage pregnancy – meanings and solutions?

When looking at the emergence of this moral panic in the 1980s, it is at first glance difficult to understand why teenage pregnancy, which had always existed, should suddenly be a social 'problem'. The concern consisted of two main elements: the question of the cost to public expenditure in the form of benefits, and the often moralistic opposition to the media-constructed figure of irresponsible and feckless young mothers who are instrumental in creating a culture of dependency. The main focus of concern was not the fact of teenage pregnancy and motherhood itself, but the fact that these young women were *unmarried* and therefore did not fit into the model of the family demanded by welfare policies. The higher rate of teenage conceptions during the 1950s and 1960s had not caused a similar panic because the majority of these ended in marriage, even if it was a 'shot-gun' one with a high propensity to end in divorce. The unmarried mother has historically been a stigmatised figure. They made up a high proportion of the inmates of the workhouses and asylums throughout the nineteenth century, were consigned to 'mother and baby' homes in the interwar and postwar period, and excluded from the Beveridge blueprint of the welfare state (Lewis 1999). Although the stigma of illegitimacy has all but disappeared from public discourse, it has been replaced by the stigma of the unmarried mother as being dependent upon state benefits and the label of 'scrounger' routinely applied. The increase in divorce has of course added to the ranks of unmarried motherhood, and although divorced mothers make up the majority of lone parents, it is still the figure of the young never-married mother that haunts public imagery and political debates. In the USA, where teenage pregnancy is highest and where the theories of the underclass and 'welfare dependency' originated, new 'tough love' measures have been taken to combat the cycle of disadvantage. The Wisconsin scheme, which has been copied by ten other states, is simple, a person can only claim five years of benefits throughout their lifetime from the age of 18. For those under 18, they must either remain at home with their parents or enter a hostel or 'Second Chance Home' but they cannot be independently allocated accommodation in social or public housing (*The Observer* 2000). At present, Britain is not contemplating adopting similar measures but the focus of government policy is firmly on the high rate of teenage pregnancy.

Britain has the highest rate of teenage pregnancy in Europe, twice that of Germany, three times that of France and six times that of the Netherlands. But despite these figures, it remains a small minority of conceptions and pregnancies; in 1997 there were 95,500 conceptions to women under twenty, including 8,300 to those under sixteen. But over half of all under-sixteen conceptions end in abortion, and the number of live births to women under twenty was 46,000 and to those under sixteen it was a mere 1,600. The main cause for concern however is revealed by the fact that only one in ten births to teenagers in 1997 took place within marriage (ONS 1997). The variation in rates between social groups and regions is also of great significance when looking for a social meaning to explain the concern. Teenage conceptions are not uniform throughout the social strata nor do they have the same outcome among various groups. For instance, the rate of terminations are much higher among the more educated and affluent. Teenage pregnancy within marriage is a norm for many within the Muslim communities. It is ironic that the traditional ideas surrounding motherhood and a mother's role is strongest in the most deprived and disadvantaged areas. Teenage pregnancy and motherhood have become one of the single biggest factors of social exclusion, why should this be and what solutions are suggested?

The Social Exclusion Unit (SEU) was given a remit in 1997 to

> develop an integrated strategy to cut rates of teenage parenthood, particularly under-age parenthood, towards the European average, and to propose better solutions to combat the risk of social exclusion for vulnerable teenage parents and their children. (SEU 1999a)

Although the Unit employs the gender-free language of 'parents', it is, of course, mothers, who are once again the focus of governmental action. Who are the teenage mothers and fathers?

The risk factors that have been isolated by the report of the Social Exclusion Unit are:

- Poverty – the risk of becoming a teenage mother is ten times higher for a girl from the unskilled manual class than from a professional family.
- Children leaving care are especially vulnerable, one survey has shown that a quarter of all care leavers had a child by the age of 16, and nearly half were mothers within 24 months of leaving care.
- Being a child of a teenage mother – the daughter of a teenage mother is twice as likely to be one herself.
- Educational underachievement – low achievement, lack of qualifications and school exclusion are all co-related with teenage parenthood.
- Sexual abuse – estimates from US studies have shown that the incidence of childhood abuse is twice as high among pregnant teenagers.
- Mental health – studies suggest a link between mental health problems and teenage pregnancy. A 1991 study found that a third of teenage girls with a conduct disorder were pregnant before the age of 17.
- Crime – it has been estimated that 25 per cent of the 11,000 teenaged boys in Young Offenders Institutions are fathers.

Teenage parenthood is clearly then both an indicator and causation of potentially lifelong social and economic disadvantage and exclusion. Intervention to tackle the problem at source and to prevent further escalation of familial disadvantage is required. The SEU published in 1999 its report and recommendations for a programme of action in *Teenage Pregnancy* (SEU 1999a). Like the other policies we have looked at, this also represents an shift from an epidemiological model to one of intervention across a wide field of activity (see Figure 6.5).

The emphasis on the role of school nurses and others in the education and support of young people tends to suppose that they are in need of information

Figure 6.5   Tackling teenage pregnancy

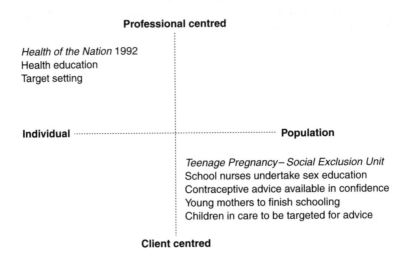

on contraception and relationships which they do not possess. But is this an accurate picture? Recent research (D. Churchill et al. 2000) suggests that this is an oversimplification and that, in their study, 93 per cent of pregnant teenagers had in fact consulted a health professional in the year previous to conception and had discussed contraception at this time and 50 per cent had in fact been prescribed oral contraception. This study further showed that those who opted for a termination were more likely to have received emergency contraception (the morning-after pill) on previous occasions.

What do these findings mean for intervention by community health professionals? It could mean that the reasons for teenage pregnancy are not simple but that many people working with young people are already in possession of invaluable insights into the meanings they give their lives. Health visitors working in projects with young people, such as sex advice centres and Sure Start programmes, for example, could be a valuable resource for research into this important issue.

There remain, however, two areas where the objective of social inclusion and restoration in the community appears to have been negated – the perennial 'outsiders' – care for the frail elderly and mental health legislation.

The perennial Cinderellas of social policy

Historically, both these groups have been the main object of community nursing care and attention. But recent policy moves have, to a degree, reformulated their position as receivers of care in the community. Concern over the cost of providing community-based and residential care to frail elderly people has dominated much of social policy thinking. The result of reports and deliberations on the future of long-term care has culminated in one of the first divisions in policy between the countries of the UK.

Shortly after their election in 1997, the New Labour government appointed a Royal Commission to 'examine the short and long term options for a sustainable system of funding of long-term care for elderly people both in their own homes and in other settings' (HMSO 1999). The Commission published the Report entitled *With Respect to Old Age* in 1999. It was a report which was controversial in that it represented a division within the Commission and the publication of both a Minority and a Majority Report. The controversy grew when the government acted upon the results of the Minority Report. There were two main recommendations of the Majority report:

- The costs of long-term care should be split between living costs, housing costs, and personal care. Personal care (which is not strictly defined as nursing care) should be available according to need and funded out of taxation.
- The establishment of a National Care Commission to monitor demography changes and spending, to set benchmarks for care provision and to represent the interests of users.

It was the matter of the funding of 'personal care' which caused the divide within the Commission, the dissenting report argued that the demand for such care would inexorably rise if it were provided free out of taxation and that this in turn would lead to an increase in costs.

The divide between the two approaches can be seen as a clear illustration of the political and philosophical divide between the 'modernisers' who see the future of funding as a partnership between public and private finance with the expectation that people who have the means must be expected to behave in a responsible way and fund their own care needs. The dissenting authors referred to the Third Way philosophy of modernisation and argued that 'old age shouldn't be seen as a time of rights without responsibilities' (HMSO 1999:116).

The Majority Report was firmly on the side of the funding of personal care out of taxation and a total rejection of any form of means testing, this version of the recommendations was put into place in Scotland but in England and Wales, personal care is to be means tested.

The problem for assessments is the definition of the constitution of personal as opposed to nursing care. For the Majority of the Commission, the term personal care denotes the 'touching of a person's body' and not living, housing, cleaning or related costs. But this is unacceptable to the dissenters who foresee a potential 'explosion' in claims. This of course has great significance for the future practice of community nursing.

Since the early 1980s when the policy of de-institutionalisation of long-stay mental patients was implemented, the plight and danger represented by released people has become a signifier of the failure of community care. Since

1997, therefore, mental health legislation has also been the subject of a modernisation agenda. As early as 1998, the government published its strategic plan for *Modernising Mental Health* services (DoH 1999) in which the then Minister of Health, Frank Dobson, stated in the Foreword 'Community Care has failed'. This Paper argued for the setting up of small specialist units for the hospital-based treatment of those deemed to be dangerous to either themselves or the public. The trend then appears to be away from community-based care and back to some form of institutionalisation and compulsion. This is illustrated in the following consultation paper *Reform of the Mental Health Act* (HMSO 2000). Although one of the main recommendations was for the provision of greater flexibility in the treatment of person with severe mental disorders, nevertheless, there was an emphasis on compulsion to treatment whether outside or inside a hospital. The protection of the public was the first priority of the provision of an improved mental health service. The paper also included a definition of mental disorder which specifically excluded sexual preference including paedophilia and the abuse of drugs and alcohol. This definition was stretched however to include the term of severe personality disorder which previously had been excluded from diagnosis and therefore treatment under the previous mental health and criminal legal legislation. There was a recognition here that the law as it stood failed to protect the public from dangerous psychopaths such as the man convicted of the violent murder of a mother and daughter in Kent in 2000. Although the compulsion element of proposed legislation has been criticised by the Royal College of Psychiatrists, this mixture of flexibility and authoritarianism with the emphasis on the public interest as opposed to the 'rights' of the users and the expertise of the providers characterises the new political philosophy. It is this move which community nurses must accommodate within their revised practice of the future. The role of community nurses is to be at the same time widened and yet limited. We now turn to examine this new role on the front-line of policy implementation.

Community nursing – on the front-line

Those community nurses at the front-line of community nursing practice, who constitute the 'avant-guard' of the profession in terms of recognising the importance of interventions that can redirect peoples' lives, are clearly demonstrating through the model of practice that they are adopting, that a new style of service is required to meet the demands of current policy. The re-emergence of social inequality and its impact upon health has provided an impetus for some community nurses to re-examine the real nature of their role, and to recognise the importance of re-awakening an approach to practice that is embedded in prevention and social care, and is positioned at the front-line of public health. In contrast, however, there are others who continue along a path of technological development, holding the view that the 'extended role of the nurse' will benefit the profession by virtue of what Dingwall described as the 'professional grandisement' of nursing (Dingwall et al. 1988), that is they believe that by increasing their technological skills they can acquire a status traditionally awarded to doctors. Recognising that some community nurses are emulating the trajectory of the medical profession, and disagreeing with Dingwall and colleagues, Walsh and Gough (1997) comment that this type of role expansion is a way in which the community nursing profession can assert itself as an entity equal to the medical profession rather than a commodity appearing on someone else's contract, as was the experience of community nurses following the implementation of the NHS and Community Care Act (DoH 1990). It is the view of these commentators that the way of opportunity lies in establishing more equal relationships with General Practitioners, so that given legislative change, nurses will be able to be taken on as equal partners in primary care practice.

As a result, it is the optimistic view of Walsh and Gough (1997:13) that the number of nurse practitioners will increase, and the numbers of nurses directly engaged in the critical tasks of diagnosis will rise. In contrast they suggest that for the remainder of community nurses, the status of commodity will remain, and with that the dominance of medical superiority and the loss of professional self direction will prevail.

Although the model of community nursing described will undoubtedly hold many attractions for clinically-orientated nurses, and will no doubt have an added value for health care managers in terms of its potential to reduce health care costs (outcome studies of such programmes demonstrate that they can achieve a substantial net savings by decreasing acute care admissions by 54 per cent, reduce hospital days by 42 per cent and cut primary care physicians' and specialists' visit costs by 37 per cent, thus achieving a 33 per cent overall cost for health care (Waszynski et al. 2000)), the fact remains that this model of community nursing is designed to support the physician in the management of high-risk patients with chronic illness, rather than to provide the kind of care which Dingwall et al. (1998) and Donzelot (1980) have described as a 'pragmatic way' of responding to problems faced by particular groups, in order that they can plan and coordinate their lives in order to survive. This is a form of care which would fulfill the policy agenda discussed earlier, it can be seen as a means of engendering responsible citizenship, and regulating society in order to improve health and social inclusion. It is the view of commentators such as Murray (1994) that inclusion of those excluded from society by virtue of single parenthood, unemployment, poor parenting, poverty and crime is an essential form of public health care which it is recognised community nurses can provide (CPHVA 1997). Although the potential of nurses to reduce health care costs through the substitution of their technical services for medical care is of high importance (Walsh and Gough 1997) and should not be denigrated, the motives and outcomes of such developments deserve to be examined rather than accepted as the only way to prevent the commodification of community nurses by more powerful players in the health care team.

First, the motive for the development of a clinical role akin to that of a medical practitioner is said by Porter (1992:724) to be the result of nurses being aware of the benefits that professional status has bestowed on other groups. Commenting that 'professionalisation was the conceptual framework which the contiguous occupation of medicine used to advance itself, with such spectacular success', it is Porter's view that 'The desire to emulate the occupational achievements of doctors seems to have blinded nurses to the fact that professions are only one form of occupation'.

He suggests that there is no reason why nursing should rigidly adhere to this path of occupational advancement. In fact, it is the view of Porter that there are very good reasons why nursing should avoid it, in that in his opinion it is not concommitant with the roles that community nurses are now encouraged to aspire to. It is concluded that what is required is for nurses to gain occupational status by ensuring that they are performing relevant and needed roles, such as public health interventions.

Discussing the above issues from a feminist perspective, Leipert (2001) suggests that the role played by the majority of females who constitute the community nursing workforce is essential to the meta paradigm concepts of public health, the development of public health nursing and public health care. Thus, the challenge for community nurses, if they are to comply with the demands of current policy is surely to ensure that their roles are needed and relevant to the performance of government strategies.

As has been shown in the first half of this chapter, individual and behavioural causes of ill health have now been rejected as the cause of widespread inequalities in health status. Instead, there is an emphasis on structural causes of ill health such as poverty, unemployment, poor housing, poor parenting, and the behavioural consequences of such factors. Recognition of these developments in health care thinking has recently stimulated the United Kingdom Central Council for Nursing Midwifery and Health Visiting (UKCC) to consult with the profession over the fact that there is much more to community nursing than the replication of medically-orientated intervention. Although there will always be a need for technological care, its narrow focus fails to target the real and primary causes of ill health such as poverty and exclusion (UKCC 2001). What then are the challenges, and more importantly what is the community nursing response, and is it equal to the need identified by those who are conscious of the far-reaching effects of social and health inequalities (Benzeval et al. 1995)?

As has already been observed, recent government health policy seeks a health rather than an illness focus, and public health is identified as a key factor in ensuring that the UK becomes a healthier and more prosperous nation. As has been seen from the last chapter, contemporary definitions of health are broad and inclusive (WHO/EURO 1984) and public health is seen as a means of improving the health of populations and reducing health inequalities between groups of the public, and is based on the rationale that the health of individuals is inextricably linked to the health of the population as a whole.

Improvements in health are hailed as a means to ensure broader societal benefits, particularly in relation to achieving the social inclusion of sectors of the population currently excluded by virtue of health or social deficits (Benzeval et al. ibid.). This challenge to enable people to live healthier lives surely mirrors the challenge to community nurses to fulfill their professional mandate to provide care in the community and to carry out primary health care interventions. These duties should involve community nurses in a pragmatic way of responding to the problems of particular groups so that members of such groups can achieve and maintain sufficient order to plan and coordinate their daily lives in order to aspire to social inclusion. As has already been discussed in Chapter 5, Dingwall and colleagues (1988) have defined such a role as a process of social control which is far from repressive or an infringement of human rights. On the contrary, it is the view of these commentators that such interventions are a necessary form of societal regulation of forces which have the potential to disrupt and destabilise society. Community nurses' involvement in such interventions offer the 'excluded' within the general population the means to return to the 'real world' and to limit the impact of 'labelling' on their lives, thereby making the caring constructs of their profession more explicit.

Recognising the timeliness of such opportunities for community nurses, the UKCC (2000:12) defined the following challenges to the profession of community nursing which have emerged from the four countries' policies;

- reducing premature deaths,
- improving health and reducing disease,
- acting on the environmental determinants of health,
- addressing inequalities in health status,
- promoting social inclusion.

These activities surely reflect the breadth of community practice across the range of promotive, preventive, interventive, rehabilitative and terminal care activities that were identified in the work of McMurray (1990) (Chapter 5). They add strength to the argument that the 'umbrella term', community nursing, encompasses a spectrum of divergent knowledge, skills and competencies, some of which bear little resemblance to the technological skills practised by the majority of medical practitioners and clinical nurse practitioners. Consideration of the rationale provided by the UKCC for involvement of health visitors and school nurses in strategies of social inclusion clearly illustrates the breadth of responsibilities that these branches of community nursing should consider if they are to rise to the challenge of policy papers such as *Our Healthier Nation* (DoH 1998a), *Better Health – Better Wales* (WO. 1998) and *Working Together for a Healthier Scotland* (SO. 1998), which all contain the universal message that poverty and exclusion are the largest causes of ill health. Such responsibilities encompass a wide range of factors that influence health and wellbeing. Some of these factors will now be addressed in order to provide examples of innovative interventions that community nurses are undertaking to improve the public health of excluded groups.

Education, training and employment

It is pointed out in the Consultation Document 'Developing standards and competencies for Health Visitors' (UKCC 2001), that there are strong connections between the physical and mental health of young people, and between their emotional health and education. Problems with family and peers are identified as important factors influencing school attendance and the capacity of young people to learn. It is quoted that some studies suggest that as many as 40 per cent of children may not be emotionally capable of taking advantage of the education that is available to them (NAfW 2000). In addition, low priority has been given to the schooling of children in care. Children, who as a consequence of the above problems may become involved in truancy, are more than three times more likely to offend than non-truants. Five per cent of all offences committed by children occur during school hours; 40 per cent of robberies, 25 per cent of burglaries and 20 per cent of criminal damage is committed by children between the ages of 10–16 years. Children who have a poor school attendance record are more likely to receive a custodial sentence than those with more positive reports. At one Young Offenders Institution, less than one in five young men (15–17 years old) had acquired the basic skills of reading, and only one in ten had the basic skills to write. The most powerful predictor of unemployment at age 21 years is non-participation in the workforce for six months or more at the age of 16–18 years. 75 per cent of males aged 16–17 who are charged in Youth Courts are not engaged in any full-time activity. In most cases the peak age for the onset of offending is 13 plus but no full-time activity substantially increases the opportunity (DfEE 1999, Social Exclusion Unit 1999). The development of a 'Connexions' Service in England aims to support and advise young people at critical points in their lives as they move through education into employment (DfEE 2000).

Extending Entitlement in Wales parallels the Connexions developments in England and aims to help every young person to realise their full potential by encouraging them to participate in education training and work. There are strong links between the health and social welfare of young children and their capacity to achieve, develop skills and contribute through work as citizens and future parents (NAfW 2000). It is recommended that health visitors and school nurses assist young people to fulfill their potential through education, skill development and participation in work schemes, thereby ensuring better health of future generations (UKCC 2001). This means that if these particular groups of community nurses accept this challenge they will be able to demonstrate the true nature of their caring role and how it differs from the medically-orientated role of others. Farrington (1995) showed that health visitors through intensive programmes of intervention have reduced school failure, child conduct problems and the incidence of juvenile crime. This example illustrates the opportunities for the polarisation of community nursing into socio-economic and medical models, each of which has a value in modern society.

Poor parenting

Poor parental supervision and lack of commitment to education by parents are crucial factors underlying truancy. There are also a number of links between child offending and parenting, such as neglect and lack of supervision, conflict between parents and children involving the child's disobedience and the parent's failure to exert control; deviant behaviour and attitudes on behalf of the parent; family disruption, in particular emotional disturbance and aggression. In addition, parental criminality is a strong predictor of delinquency and persistent offending. The Sure Start programmes in England, Wales and Northern Ireland and the Children's Services Plans and Family Centres in Scotland, often organised by health visitors, are all aimed at ensuring that children growing up in families with few resources are offered support from an early age to give them the best start in life through promoting their development (Home Office 1998, Scottish Executive 1999, Youth Justice Board 1999). Sutton has shown how professional support from health visitors, school nurses and practice nurses can provide the necessary parenting education for families experiencing difficulties (Health Visitor 1995), thereby bringing such families 'in from the cold' rather than coercing them to change their behaviour.

Community safety and crime prevention

In Welsh prisons, 40 per cent of offenders are under 25, most are likely to be both victims and perpetrators of crime, and most are likely to have had some experience of the care system. A review of young prisoners (HMIP 1997) indicated that 40 per cent of young people in custody reported having a long standing illness – almost double the figure for the general population. Over 50 per cent of young prisoners on remand and 30 per cent of sentenced young offenders have a diagnosable mental disorder, 84 per cent of young prisoners aged 16–24 were current smokers averaging 13 cigarettes a day, 94 per cent had drunk alcohol, 37 per cent had drunk heavily and 86 per cent had used drugs. The Audit Commission describes what it terms a cycle of antisocial behaviour, comprising of inadequate parenting, aggressive or hyperactive behaviour, truancy or exclusion, peer group pressure, unstable living conditions, lack of training and employment, drug and alcohol abuse, with poor parenthood itself closing the circle. The WHO suggests that there may be a significant overlap between factors associated with antisocial behaviour and those which give rise to the problems of ill health. Hence, action by community nurses towards improving one dimension of such behaviours may have a beneficial influence on the others (NAfW 2000, NACRO 1999). Farrington (ibid.) recommends that it would be cost effective in the light of the success of health visiting intervention to reduce juvenile crime, to re-allocate a proportion of the criminal justice budget to provide intensive health visiting programmes for high-risk families (Farrington 1995).

Drug taking

71 per cent of those out of education, employment or training have used drugs as opposed to 47 per cent of their peers. School truants are twice as likely to have tried solvents of illicit drugs and three times more likely to have tried hard drugs as non-truants. Those involved with drugs are more likely to be offenders (NAfW 2001, Scottish Executive 1999). The Acheson Report (DoH 1998b) showed how school-based interventions could prevent substance misuse. Community nurses, particularly school nurses and community psychiatric nurses, are well placed to provide interventive services for this group.

Safeguarding and promoting the rights of children and young people

49 per cent of young women prisoners report having been sexually abused, and 39 per cent had children (DoH 1998, HMPS 1997). The Strategy for Children and Young People in Wales emphasises the need for preventive services that allow people to get help and advice without stigma. This draws on the consensus that many of the problems which become serious in adolescence could have been mitigated by better, and more responsive, services for younger children, greater attention to the contribution of play, and other enriching opportunities for people's health wellbeing and attainment (NAfW 2000). These considerations of the interplay between health and social disadvantage illustrate that the government's interest in joined-up services through public health intervention could result in considerable cost savings in health care. Indeed calculations of potential savings categorically show that this is undoubtedly the case. It has been shown that many of the needs of children and young people are currently being met by various community nursing disciplines, and the need for increasing such interventions obviously exists. Yet, the declining numbers of health visitors and school nurses (Clark et al. 2000) must surely pose a threat to the likelihood of this occurring, and consequently a threat to social inclusion, responsible families, modernisation, equity and public health. Finally, however, it is argued that expansion of the public health role of community nurses as evidenced above cannot fail to expose the construction of the profession of community nursing as one that is concerned as

much with care as it is with cure. Review of current activities of community nurses helps to substantiate this claim, the literature shows that community nurses are already making a large contribution to the delivery of primary care and community services for public health. The CPHVA (2000) stated that community nurses are very well aware of those groups in society who have been disenfranchised in terms of accessibility to services, such groups include ethnic minorities, the homeless, travellers and victims of domestic violence as well as the many others discussed above. Claims that the profession of community nursing has a common ideological base (UKCC 1994) therefore have to be questioned, and the desire to mould community nurses into a flexible commodity model of care provision should be carefully reconsidered if both socio-economic and medical care interventions are required.

The Review of Health Visiting and School Nursing in Wales (Clark et al. 2000) showed that health visitors working in Health Action Zones have founded post-natal depression groups with creches to care for children; health visitors and school nurses are also looking after the health needs of young offenders within Youth Offending Teams; Sure Start schemes for areas of deprivation and high ethnic minority populations are also managed by health visitors and midwives; school nurses and health visitors are also working with prisoners and their families. In Wales again, the CPHVA has shown that a specialist interest group from within its membership has carried out a research project in to the health and living conditions of homeless families. This work clearly highlighted the emotional distress of homeless adults; the effects of homelessness on the healthy development of children which commonly arose from a lack of play space; the fact that poor housing seriously disadvantages families in that the majority of such families had little or no facilities for the storage, preparation, and cooking of food; 85 per cent of families were shown to be living in unsafe and unhealthy environments. Health visitors involved in this research are working in housing projects in urban and rural areas throughout England. In addition to their work on homelessness, health visitors have also drawn attention to the importance of quality, choice and design in housing provision. Particularly, they have criticised the housing of young families in upper-floor flats and maisonettes without controlled entry or lifts, saying that they are not acceptable homes for the following reasons. Parents with small children are faced daily with the dilemma of whether to leave the baby, the toddler or the shopping at the bottom of an open stairway. People whose mobility is compromised or who suffer sensory impairment or serious debilitating illness have the same problems. Level access, turning space, wide doors and lifts are required for prams, pushchairs and wheelchairs. These facilities could be incorporated into the design of flats thus eliminating the need for rehousing on health grounds. Alderman (2000) and Aurora and Irvine (2000) have shown that community nurses are providing valuable contributions to the development and functioning of Health Improvement Programmes (HIPs) and Primary Care Groups (PCGs) in London and Bradford thereby illustrating the positive effects of social interaction on health. Clendon and White

(2001) evaluated the effectiveness of a school-based parenting programme run by community nurses; their findings show that parents benefited from the programme by gaining a sense of control over the parental role, an increased ability to empathise with their children, the capacity to think about matters calmly and to reduce unhelpful parenting practices such as shouting and smacking. Northumbria Health Care Trust has shown how community nurses have developed a parenting project that will lead to thematic collaborative and consistent parenting activity across all agencies both statutory and voluntary. The group have been highly productive and have made great steps in promoting cross-agency working. Daniel (2000) has shown how a health visitor and a district nurse working collaboratively have addressed the issue of men's health in Warrington, a place synonymous with the tough, professional sport of rugby league, and a propensity to ignore important health issues because of cultural beliefs. Similarly, Chell (2000) has shown how community nurses in the Bradford and Airdale region have provided programmes to eliminate inequalities in men's health.

There are many accounts of community nursing programmes organised and managed by health visitors and school nurses, a fact which fires the notion that, of necessity, the nature of this form of practice is firmly embedded in a socio-economic model of health care, which can be contrasted with the ways in which other caring interventions are carried out. As is shown in Chapter 7, this does not mean that the practice of health visitors and school nurses is of more or less value, merely that it is a different form of care. District nurses are also making a valuable contribution to improvements in community care. Mooney and Symonds (2001) showed how the services of district nurses were crucial to the smooth functioning of 'day care services' for people requiring surgery for varicose veins and hernias. In this qualitative study of patients who had recently experienced day care surgery, it was shown that increased involvement of district nurses prior to surgical intervention could speed up the process of recovery. A.M. Jones (2000), in a study of the barriers between health and social care, showed how district nursing services were vital to the care of the chronic sick. Thus, it is apparent from recent reviews of community nursing care that community nurses are providing a wide range of social and health interventions, they are concerned with both cure and care, and both aspects of these polarised interventions need equity. It would appear from the evidence presented that community nurses are already placing a much greater emphasis on improving health through community-based approaches, intersectoral activity, environmental interventions, health promotion activities, disease prevention programmes and the provision of essential curative care. However, tensions still persist in respect of determining the real nature of community nursing roles. It would appear that continued reluctance to recognise the need for a broad range of community nursing interventions is affecting the image of the profession.

Constructions of community nursing which only emphasise clinical skills serve only to tarnish the caring image of nursing. As has been stated by Malone

(2002), the General Secretary of the RCN in the United Kingdom, 'The wake-up call to nurses is to ensure that they can confidently articulate the nature of the care that they provide'.

The evidence to support the value of social care as a means of improving health status is legion, some individual groups of community nurses have, of necessity, to be different if interventions across a spectrum of care both health and social are to be valued. To create a valued and successful image, community nurses should be celebrating their different skills, and enunciating the ways in which their skills can be used collaboratively to improve public health. Thereby a spectrum of care needs can be fulfilled and the public can be assured that their needs for health and social wellbeing will be met effectively.

Conclusion

The purpose of this chapter has been to discuss three main issues, the current direction and meaning of policies concerned with the restoration of community and social inclusion; the vulnerable groups at which policy is directed, and the real lived experience of community nurses and health visitors in the front-line of care provision. It was shown how, despite a continuation of private enterprise management goals in health care, there is at the centre of policy a desire to tackle social exclusion and to restore community and that this has activated a revival of concern about public health, as evidenced by the appointment of a minister for public health. This perceived shift in policy has created opportunities for an enhanced role for community nurses and health visitors in that social as well as health care interventions are required, and the targeting of vulnerable groups and communities demands a much broader focus of nursing and public health practice. The persistence of health inequalities, despite over half a century of a health service 'free' at the point of delivery indicates that community nursing interventions, based on *individual* and 'blaming the victim' approaches to the management of 'lifestyle disease' have ignored the structural causes of ill health. Thus, the failure of community nurses, particularly health visitors and school nurses, to engage in wider campaigns for the improvement of community health, because of medical and managerial restraints on models of practice, has resulted in an increasing emphasis on medical models of intervention, and a weakened focus and understanding of the real meaning of the concept of care.

However, it has been shown that more recent policy has focused on the fact that poverty is the single largest cause of ill health and, as a result, the solutions to health care problems have become more varied and increasingly diverse in respect of the knowledge and skills required to address structural inequalities, and improve health and wellbeing. The discourses of these policies, social inclusion, work, responsible families and modernisation in health and social care, have created new opportunities for community nurses to change the culture of nursing care, and thereby to increase public responsibility for the planning and controlling of every-day life. The opportunity for community nurses to exercise social control through appropriate forms of health care intervention such as support, and empowerment strategies means that the public opportunity to receive a positive experience from health care interventions is enhanced. Several examples of this kind of service provision are provided, and it is concluded that for community nurses there is an increasing divide between the demands of public social interventionist skills and practice to solve 'social problems' which impact on health status, and the demands for skills and practice competency to fulfill the demands of 'private' and individually-orientated home-based nursing care. Community nursing is therefore being separated by policy aims into its various component parts that have been described as prevention, promotion, intervention, rehabilitation and terminal care. It is concluded that each branch of community nursing; health visitors, school nurses, learning disability nurses, mental health nurses, district nurses, and palliative care nurses all have an important contribution to make to public health, but that the nature of each of these roles should be celebrated for its uniqueness and difference, rather than criticised for its recalcitrancy to blur itself into an oblivion of conformity to a common generic role.

Summary

In this chapter we have been concerned to analyse the meaning and direction of policies aimed at tackling social exclusion and active citizenship. In contrast to the preceding years, since 1997 policies have been focused more on the population or communities rather than on individuals. This represents a challenge to community nursing practice as, historically, the individual or family have been the main focus of attention.

Targets on tackling health inequalities require a 'joined-up' approach with multi-agency working and especially the expansion of the role of health visiting and social work. In many ways the emphasis on the community is for health visiting, a return to an earlier tradition of 'working on the patch' rather than a case work approach.

The shift towards a new way of defining and organizing welfare services is based upon a redefinition of citizens. The ideal of the active citizen is one who participates fully in the life of their community and is part of a wider communitarian culture. Access to employment is the passport to benefits and services for everyone including mothers with school-aged children. This is a new direction for policies and has at its heart the person of the 'universal worker'. The gendered identities of mother and father have become subsumed under the generic description of 'parents'. Potentially this marks a break in the assumption of health visiting as being primarily concerned with mothers and babies at home.

Community nurses are being required to return to their roots in public health and community development in a wider sense.

CHAPTER 7

Reconstructing an Image for the Twenty-first Century

Introduction

Towards the end of the 1990s, government White Papers on Health (DoH 1997, WO 1998) signalled a shift in the focus of health care provision away from services provided in hospitals towards preventive care services provided in community settings. Frameworks for health care provided by this policy devolved the responsibility for identification of health and social care needs, and the provision of services to a local level, making Primary Care Groups (England), Local health Groups (Wales) and Local Health Boards (Scotland) responsible for planning and delivering services responsive to people's needs. An emphasis on the importance of collaborative care raised the hopes of community nurses that the focus on medically-orientated cure would give way to a care-orientated model of intervention, and that they would have at last an opportunity to move away from the oppression of medical and managerial domination of their roles. However, guidance as to the composition of collaborative PHC structures soon made it plain that medical domination had not been weakened. Whereas representation of nurses was stipulated in these documents together with local authority, health authority, pharmacist, dental practitioner, optometrist representation and lay people, these representatives were far outweighed by the number of doctors that could be appointed. These developments have led sceptics to comment that the nursing contribution to health and social wellbeing is not valued or understood by other professionals or even by nurses themselves (Vaughan 1999). As a result, community nurses are still prevented from constructing an image of themselves that conveys the philosophical nature of their profession and from autonomously exercising care based on their specific expertise and knowledge. Agreeing with this view, Lyne (1997) suggests that the problem relates to nurses' inability to communicate their contribution to care. The solution to this problem does not, in Lyne's view, lie in the expansion of nursing roles into the medical domain, a response that nurses appear to be making through, for example, the development of nurse practitioner and advanced practitioner roles (Kelly 1998). On the contrary, Lyne (ibid.) suggests that the only solution lies in an articulation of the essence of nursing (care) and its application to a health system built on social concepts of health and wellbeing. To construct a new image and take advantage of the opportunities which present themselves in the shape of current policy, Lindsey and Harrick (1996) suggest that nurses need to achieve more control over nursing work and they should seek to influence health goals. However, despite the fact that it is the contention of nursing literature (Klainberg and colleagues 1998) that no profession is better qualified, or as well placed as community nursing to implement the new policy agenda, there are many outside of the profession that are still unable or unwilling to recognise the potential contribution that nurses could make to improving primary health care. Though, as the previous chapter has shown, there is evidence to show that community nursing forays into the realms of community development for health are beginning to demonstrate the value of community nursing as a profession which is able to assist the process of social control through caring interventions aimed at mitigating undesirable social circumstances. In this chapter, there will be a discussion of how community nurses can redefine their image, the barriers that they will encounter in so doing and of current constructs of community nursing and decision-making in terms of constructing a 'new image'. It is argued that, to convey the real nature of community nursing, the need for collective public health interventions must be made explicit, and the diversity of interventions catalogued through the processes of research and evaluation. Only by convincing politicians, managers and doctors of the broad remit of community nursing care, and the vast range of nursing responsibilities can the chains of governmentality be finally discarded. To respond to current policy challenges, community nurses have a public responsibility to show that the divergence of need in community settings requires a divergence in the focus of nursing care. Health cannot be attained by a mere 'medical' focus of intervention, the provision of social support is a form of social control which can achieve social inclusion.

Redefining the identity of community nursing

To redress the situation wherein the real nature of community nursing is poorly understood, and the role of community nurses is continually refined by others through the process of governmentality, McMurray (1990) suggests that community nurses must recommit, redefine and re-polish their professional identity by adopting a role which links professional, political and social advocacy as convergent strategies for community empowerment and development. Agreeing with this view, Macleod Clark (1993) suggests that a change in the philosophy of nursing is needed, away from medically-influenced clinical interventions towards a more client-orientated approach, which could be achieved through supporting and facilitating care rather than imposing clinical interventions. As Macdonald (1992) has pointed out, medical models of care are obstacles to people's participation in health and social care, it is no longer possible to simply tell the community what is wrong with their health, as was typically the model of intervention used in health promotion during the 1980s (see Chapter 6). Successful intervention is, in Macdonald's opinion, dependent on community involvement in future planning. However, Bamford (1990) has suggested that whilst nurses continue to battle against a legacy of domination fuelled by gender discrimination (Davies 1995), the way forward will not be easy. What is required is that nurses demonstrate that 'caring' is 'work' and that this is a form of work that does not make them subservient.

Historical barriers to the construction of a new image

Dingwall and colleagues (1988) remind us that the answers to current problems sometimes lie in the past. Therefore, to shed some light on the current ambivalences in the constructs of community nursing, some of the historical events underlying its development will be revisited. Even from the earliest days of the profession the ambivalence between the curing and caring roles of nurses was identified as a contentious issue. Nightingale, for example, in her 'Notes on Nursing' (1859) demonstrated her hostility to hospital-based health care by giving priority to preventive work. In Dingwall's view, this early text on nursing was one of the first in the creation of what Armstrong (1983:7–8) called the Dispensary, a metaphor for the conceptual shift which has extended medicine from the correction of the sick in segregated and regulated institutions, to the social control of the healthy (Figure 7.1). For Nightingale, community nursing was a civilising occupation aimed at reforming and redirecting the lives of people, not just caring for them (see Chapter 6). In her view, the philanthropic delivery of care in the absence of a more rigorous and coordinated approach to improve social and economic behaviour was a waste of effort. A rigorous approach to community nursing was therefore advised, where the backgrounds and needs of those requiring a service would be scientifically measured and their compliance with prescriptions for social and economic behaviour carefully monitored. Those that rejected the standards demanded would, in Nightingale's opinion, forfeit expectations for care. This is a kind of social discipline which bears resemblance to the contemporary need for an inclusive society (Oppenheim and Harker 1996) and characterises the 'Third Way' policy forwarded by New Labour (see Chapter 6). As Nightingale saw it, the role of the community nurse was to instil social discipline as well as to care. In her view this philosophy created a need for workers possessing high moral character, recruits from a higher social class, and more rigorous training. Nightingale constantly underlined the differences between nursing inside hospital, where there is an elaborate system of discipline and control to structure nurses work, and nursing in the home (or community) where the nurse has to rely on her personal qualities and skills. Indeed, Nightingale went as far as to assert that 'The District Nurse must... be of yet higher class and of yet fuller training than a hospital nurse' (Nightingale 1876, quoted from Baly 1986:128). Similarly in relation to health visitors

Nightingale, in her correspondence with the Chairman of the North Buckingham Technical Education Committee, Frederick Verney, wrote, 'It hardly seems necessary to contrast sick nursing with [health visiting]... [the health visitor] must create a new work and a new profession for women'.

Commenting on the way in which these views found a practical expression in the work of community nurses, Donzelot (1980:82–95) described the benefits of a 'tutelary relationship' which nurses could build between families and the state. However, it would appear that philosophical debate underpinning the exact nature of community nursing work has still to be resolved as, throughout the years, the core issues underlying the debate such as the nature of care and the relevance of social control have been subservient to discussion of education and management issues. Consequently it is these latter factors that appear to have had the most influence on the development of the professions.

Education and the development of community nursing

Developments in nurse education can be viewed as part of a continuing struggle between professional and managerial constructs of the occupation of nursing. Dingwall et al. (1988) suggest that throughout the history of the development of the nursing profession there has been ambivalence between a utilitarian emphasis on service provision and attempts to 'gentrify' the occupation by raising its status to that of the medical profession. According to Dingwall, radical reform of nurse education began with the Briggs Report (HMSO 1972) which set out to resolve the poor image of nursing held by school leavers in order to attract better-qualified entrants. Proposals were for a nursing curriculum structured along medical lines, with a general foundation leading on to specialist education. Although the proposals represented an apparent egalitarian system of education, potentially, they created a meritocracy in nursing through a series of awards for continuing programmes of study. (Dingwall et al. 1988). The proposed content of training reformulated the objective of Nightingale to integrate curative and preventive work, but appeared to ignore the philosophical focus of nursing interventions and the differing responsibilities of hospital and community nurses that had been noted by Nightingale. To oversee this system, Briggs (ibid.) proposed the consolidation of the various bodies responsible for pre- and post-registration training in all of the various specialities and parts of the UK. It was suggested that a single powerful Council supported by National Boards would be responsible for bringing all sections of the occupation under its governance and implementing policies and discipline. Thus, the specific nature of various parts of the profession in terms of duties related to care and/or control were ignored. The only specialty to retain some autonomy was midwifery which was to be regulated by a statutory committee of the Council (HMSO 1972:185–90).

Although the recommendations of Briggs were finally introduced in November 1978, the reforms concentrated on changes of regulatory structures rather than educational requirements and ignored the fundamental nature of nursing work. Despite the insistence of these recommendations that nursing should be seen as a profession equal to but separate from medicine (HMSO 1972:158), various specialist interests such as community nurses feared that the concentration of power would lead to ideological dominance of clinical intervention. The benefit of hindsight shows that these fears have indeed been realised, as during the 1970s the recommendations of the Briggs Report facilitated the priorities of the DHSS to bring about successive reorganisations of the NHS, and achieve closer integration of hospital and community-based services, thereby increasing the reliance on clinical or technological care in community settings, such as the health centre or the home. Thus, it can be seen that the reform of nurse education may have been dominated more by the need for improved management of the NHS, particularly in respect of the rationalisation of resources, rather than a concern to develop the profession. Integration of curative and preventive branches of the nursing profession through the establishment of one regulatory body provided government with the means of creating a more effective and efficient use of physical resources and a more flexible workforce. Thus, the Nurses, Midwives and Health Visitors' Act (1979) can be interpreted as a great disappointment in the history of the development of nursing, particularly community nursing. As Dingwall et al. (1988) show, instead of the construction of a new licence for autonomous practice that the Act could have conferred, it merely provided low-cost administrative reform and, but for concessions which had to be made to a number of special interest groups, such as health visitors who were allowed to maintain their registerable status, and midwives who were allowed to maintain their own committee, it gave the Council licence to impose a unified view of the occupation's status and direction. Far from being a view which enhanced the philosophical ideals of all branches of nursing, this was a view which again emphasised the subservience of nursing to medical and managerial influences and provided a precedent for further educational reform.

Project 2000 (1986) strengthened the analogy with medical education by envisaging new nurse practitioners who would be flexible, knowledgeable and able to work within a variety of settings both in the hospital and the community. Although this new system of education separated nurse education from nursing services, and was revolutionary in terms of its intentions to create more autonomous practitioners, well versed in clinical decision-making and professional judgement (Dingwall et al. 1988), it created a single level of registered nurse who, although orientated towards the provision of health care to the community and versed in the prevention of ill health and primary health care in line with the World Health Organisation (1986) recommendations and those of the European Conference on Nursing (1988), its main focus on clinical care appeared to limit the debate on the philosophical focus of nursing intervention, particularly in community settings. It would therefore appear that educational programmes which had been designed to improve the status of nurses were still failing to enable nurses to articulate the essence of nursing and its application to a health system built on social concepts of health and wellbeing for all. As a result, it would appear that the caring side of nursing may have become devalued, or overlooked by increasingly well-educated practitioners who perceive there is more 'kudos' to be gained from being at the 'sharp' end of clinical nursing interventions. As a result, there are reports, such as those of Takase and colleagues (2000) of increasing image discrepancies between the public and nurses, regarding community nursing. According to these commentators, although it has long been recognised that nurses live in a dual structure wherein their journey towards professionalisation has been constrained by stereotypes held by society, failure to address this discrepancy will continue to meet with public disapproval, and will reduce nurses self-concept, job satisfaction and performance. It is their belief that, only by improving the current public image of nursing can the professionalisation of nursing be enhanced. Agreeing with this view, Chen and colleagues (2001) showed that the ideal image of a nurse is based more on ability to provide emotional support, comfort, correct information and advice, and advocacy than on the provision of technical interventions exclusively. This suggests that the present government's emphasis on the need to 'bring back matrons' (DoH 2000) may not be a strategy that is too wide of the mark, if the intention of this move is to improve standards of care.

Management and the development of community nursing

Throughout the 1970s, the DHSS was concerned with the desire to reform the health services, and in keeping with a contemporary fashion in management theory, reform was achieved through processes of central planning and bureaucratisation. According to Dingwall et al. (1988), in the NHS a collegial form of bureaucracy was adopted in the guise of 'consensus management' and as a result nurses, as representatives of a major professional group, were invited to join administrators in developing rational plans for the development of the services input. Part of this process was in Dingwall's view apparently designed to encourage nurses to become key allies of the administrators in the control of the medical professions, as nurses were seen as substitutes for medical labour and lower-cost solutions for many of the expenditure problems of the NHS. However, according to Robinson and Strong (1987:22–9), nurse managers failed to grasp the critical issues of service policy and planning, and many obstructed the development of autonomous practice by registered nurses. As a result, nurses again became subject to traditions of hierarchy and obedience, but this time subjugation operated in a modern industrial discipline under the auspices of a newly emerging form of NHS managerialism (Symonds and Kelly 1998).

By the 1980s, the outcomes of the Griffiths Inquiry into NHS Management (DHSS 1983) had encouraged the development of a more aggressive style of management focused on market orientations of care provision, and concerns for cost savings, labour inputs, purchasing and providing of services, and speed in decision-making rather than the building of consensus. Against this background, managers' interest in nursing reform was inevitable. As has been seen in previous chapters, nursing salaries constituted a large portion of public expenditure, savings therefore equated with high impacts on budgets and consequently any nursing innovation was carefully assessed for cost implication. The shift towards primary and community care during the 1980s therefore led to an emphasis on the need for increased flexibility in care, and often the care of previously institutionalised groups in community settings. As a result, community nurses were urged by the Cumberlege Report (DHSS 1986) to recognise that many problems were created by 'separate and traditional ways of working'. Following the publication of this report there was a suggestion that community nurse roles should be merged and training unified, a dictate that came to pass in relation to the education and training of specialist community nurses (UKCC 1991). However, this suggestion, and its subsequent implementation paid little heed to the different nature of nursing interventions provided by the variety of various professional groups of community nursing, and no attention was given to the differing requirements of public health and curative care. Reform of the NHS, therefore, has undoubtedly had a marked effect on all professionals who work in the service (Symonds and Kelly 1998). As the ideology driving reform has been fuelled by the need for rationalisation of health service provision, it is not too surprising to find that developments in community nursing have been limited to those which enhance cost savings or constitute substitution for medical care, rather than developments which would make the focus of nursing interventions more explicit. Thus the two community nursing roles which have seen the most development during the 1990s, are those of the nurse practitioner and the practice nurse (Littlewood 1995). In contrast, community nurses concerned with the provision of social care such as district nurses, health visitors, school nurses, and learning disability nurses have seen their roles seriously eroded (Symonds and Kelly 1998). Discourses encompassing the notion of the extended role of the nurse (Birch 2001) are couched in terms of the benefits that accrue from a realisation of how doctors' and nurses' roles can complement each other, but in reality these discourses merely disguise the emphasis that is placed on the need for an extended role to encompass technological interventions previously limited to doctors. This type of discourse therefore disguises from both nurses and the public that nursing is being constructed as a cheaper form of medical care.

Current constructs of community nursing

In an article 'Old Wine in New Bottles', Clark (2000) suggests that the new 'bottle' of community nursing holds 'plenty of wine', but people will not be carried away with the label or advertisements, what matters is what is inside.

In Clark's view, nurses must move forward into the technologically-orientated world of the twenty-first century, but at the same time they must take care not to lose the important constants, presumably the provision of care and support, that people value and need. Whilst this may be admirable advice, it has been seen from the last chapter that because of nurses' readiness to comply with medical and managerial constructs of their role, and to commit themselves to compliance with the demand for flexible care provision, they may again be being moulded into a construct of the profession devised by others rather than one of their own making. Currently, a construct of the community nurse as a technological care manager is one which does not appear to be meeting the needs or approval of client groups, as was shown by S. Jones (2000) and Sumner and Sumner (2000) in Chapter 5. Such pointers, together with the almost daily round of media criticisms of nursing care provision (albeit the criticisms are largely based on the lack of human and technical resources) alert us to the fact that the construct of the community nurse as a caring professional may be waning. As was noted by Radsma (1994), although unquestionably caring is at the root of nursing, that caring is the essence of nursing has still to be determined. It is her view that nursing as a profession cannot continue to hide behind the discourse of care without explicit and implicit understanding of what professional caring entails. It will not suffice in future to pay lip service to caring, if caring is a nursing value it must be incorporated into the socialisation of nurses. In Radsma's opinion, if nurses wish to construct themselves as a caring profession then they must ensure that the resources required to support that behaviour are also made available. In a provocative style Radsma, quoting Roach (1991), states that 'when we cease to care, we cease to be human' and asks the question 'If nurses cease to care, do they cease to be nurses?'

Such considerations obviously are of immense importance to the future of the nursing profession but, at a time of rapid change in policy and health and social care provision, it may not be surprising that nurses have little time to contemplate the nature of the image that they would wish to present to the public at large. At a time when, as a result of primary health care and community care strategy (DoH 1990), people are coming out of hospital at a faster and faster rate in sicker and sicker conditions, and the rate of socially induced illness is growing (Benzeval, Judge and Whitehead 1995), the effort to keep pace with current developments may mean that the community nursing profession is insufficiently aware of the importance of the 'public image' that it is portraying. The Audit Commission Review (1999) of district nursing services in the UK showed, for instance, that as a result of 'pressure on services to increase efficiency, and the rise in technical, as opposed to personal, nursing care, there is a danger that some of the things that patients say they value most highly from nursing will be lost'.

As the provision of palliative and terminal care at home becomes more and more common place, increasingly, because of resourcing difficulties, more and more care is being delegated to lesser-qualified staff (Griffiths 2001). It will surely become more and more difficult then for community nurses to construct a caring image, when they are no longer providing the sort of care appreciated by the public. Taking an optimistic view, however, Clark (2000) shows how care can still be delivered at a distance. Providing the example of NHS Direct, a 24-hour nurse-operated telephone service, launched by the Secretary for Health on the 5 July 1998, and quoting from the *Daily Express* (1999:16), Clark describes the outcome of a telephone consultation between a nurse and patient which resulted in the patient being admitted to hospital: ' "It was like having an invisible hand to hold", the patient said'.

Clark asserts that surely in an age when marriages are made over the Internet, people can develop relationships over the telephone. Putting flippancy aside, Clark does recognise that patient assessment and diagnosis are much more difficult when visual clues are absent and, that for this form of new technology to work, nurses will require new highly developed skills of clinical judgement over and above those that are concerned with the use of algorithmic software, such as pre-formulated frameworks of 'Nursing Diagnosis' (Carpenito 1993). As yet, there is little data available on the clinical outcomes of such care, and no audit has been carried out on the incidence of change in pre-existing conditions as a result of telephone interventions. Neither has any specific preparation been given to nurses who carry out such practice, despite the fact that they are similarly accountable for their practice as other nurses, and require similar levels of clinical supervision. Perhaps positive assessments of distanced caring should be made with caution. Over and above these considerations, and questioning the extent to which the current construction of community nursing is of a caring profession, it is salutary to recognise that there is already pressure from finance-driven managers for nurses to accept the use of algorithm-based decision-making tools as they reduce the need for expertise and facilitate 'getting away' with the lowest possible and, therefore, cheapest grade of nurse. Is this not an indication, then, that nursing is still being moulded by 'interested others' to perform intrusive tasks aimed at maintaining social order, rather than being allowed to perform enabling tasks of social control, as defined by Dingwall and colleagues (1988)? Indeed, the potential of current technological systems to impose a Foucauldian model of surveillance and control is evidenced in criticisms of contemporary services found in health care literature. For example, Florin and Rosen (1999:5) in an editorial of the *British Medical Journal* (July 1999) drew attention to the need to be wary of NHS Direct. In their view, the system typifies tensions between the conflicting goals of consumer responsiveness and 'demand management', the latest euphemism for rationing of health care, and weapon for cost containment in the NHS. GPs, at their annual conference in June 1999 showed adamant opposition to such schemes as NHS Direct, as it is seen as challenging their roles. Whilst it may be the case that this antagonism on the part of medical practitioners should be interpreted as a form of resistance to the usurping of their 'power' systems by nurses, it is just as feasible that doctors are protesting about the way in which such systems undermine their professional judgement and decision-making, and have the potential to de-professionalise them to the status of workers, a modern phenomenon noted by McKinlay and Arches (1985) in their proletarianisation thesis. If the latter supposition holds credibility the question of why nurses are prepared to 'go along' with such systems must be asked? Do such interventions enhance the public image of community nursing, or do they substitute technological intervention for care and support?

Making decisions

Considerations such as those above seriously challenge the profession of community nursing to consider carefully whether it wishes to re-establish the focus on care, which was prevalent in the early days of the profession, or whether it wishes to maintain its current emphasis on technical and procedural elements of practice. Given the direction of current health care policy (UKCC 2001) (see Figure 7.1), the time has surely come to ask the question, What is the specific focus of community nursing? Is nursing an increasingly technologically-orientated profession, which is gradually being flattered and groomed to undertake more of the territory once occupied by doctors at a much reduced cost, or is it so broad that the only way it can make itself understood, is for it to be fragmented in order that attention can be given to the more obvious and tacit aspects of the role, such as the technical and procedural elements, inherited or bountifully bestowed by reluctant others?

It is the contention of the arguments forwarded in this chapter that these questions can only be given the consideration they deserve if the latter view is adopted. To understand the real nature of community nursing and the role that it is currently challenged to fulfill by government policy, Sutton and Smith (1995) suggest that nurses should concentrate on the essence of the nurse–client relationship. In the case of community nurses, it is suggested that the essence of the nurse–client relationship spans a two dimensional axis. Thus following Beattie (1993) (Figure 7.2), the nature of community nursing can be made explicit by realising that on a horizontal axis the focus of care passes from the individual to the collective. That is, at any one time, in order to address the problems created by social determinants of health there is a need to understand that the individual's condition is relative to the collective experience. Thus, intervention at a collective level may be the best way to limit individual disease. Similarly intervention at the individual level may be the only way of recognising the effects of problems occurring at a collective level. Similarly, and simultaneously on a vertical axis, there is a spectrum of interventions which span a gradient between Authoritative (curative/technological) interventions and Negotiated (caring/preventive interventions), thus the spectrum of interventions on offer can be tailored to meet both the needs of the sick and the well population. This construct of community nursing clearly articulates the description of community nursing given by McMurray (1990:8) which

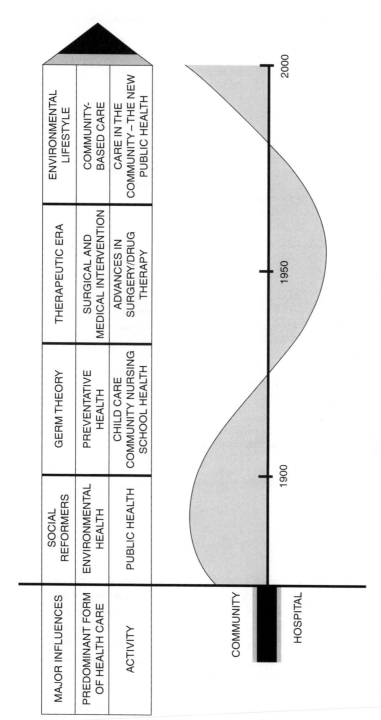

MAJOR INFLUENCES	SOCIAL REFORMERS	GERM THEORY	THERAPEUTIC ERA	ENVIRONMENTAL LIFESTYLE
PREDOMINANT FORM OF HEALTH CARE	ENVIRONMENTAL HEALTH	PREVENTATIVE HEALTH	SURGICAL AND MEDICAL INTERVENTION	COMMUNITY-BASED CARE
ACTIVITY	PUBLIC HEALTH	CHILD CARE COMMUNITY NURSING SCHOOL HEALTH	ADVANCES IN SURGERY/DRUG THERAPY	CARE IN THE COMMUNITY – THE NEW PUBLIC HEALTH

COMMUNITY

HOSPITAL

1900   1950   2000

Figure 7.1 The changing focus of health care

Figure 7.2   The scope of community nursing practice

Source: Beattie (1993)

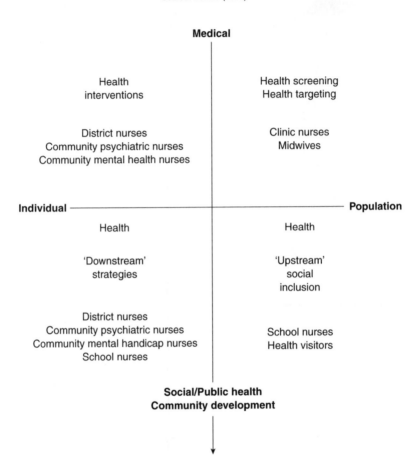

Medical

Health
interventions

Health screening
Health targeting

District nurses
Community psychiatric nurses
Community mental health nurses

Clinic nurses
Midwives

Individual ———————————————————————— **Population**

Health

'Downstream'
strategies

Health

'Upstream'
social
inclusion

District nurses
Community psychiatric nurses
Community mental handicap nurses
School nurses

School nurses
Health visitors

Social/Public health
Community development

states that

> Community health nursing is much more than nursing practised in the community setting. It is the practice of simultaneously considering and enabling the health care needs of individuals, families aggregates (population subgroups) and the total community. This demands both a clinical and public health focus of care ... Guided by a humanitarian approach, the nurse attempts to intervene with individuals and families in ways that are culturally considerate, humanely committed and responsive ... At the same time, the health needs of various subgroups and the collective needs of the population must also be considered. Additionally, there must be on going consideration of the influence of environmental factors (physical, biological, and socio-cultural) on the health of all members of the population.

The humanitarian approach must therefore be accompanied by a functional orientation that considers alternative strategies which are operational, consistent with humane and ethical views, dictated by health needs and cost effective. To practise in such a broad role, the nurse must be skilful at problem-solving, decision-making, researching, consulting, planning, organising, managing, co-ordinating, advocating, educating, counselling, providing care, referring and evaluating, as well as skilful in technological interventions.

The community health nurse is further described by McMurray (1990:10) as one whose care-giving at primary secondary and tertiary levels of primary health care intervention is guided by four concepts of practice;

- conservation – maintaining health status and preserving function,
- prevention – ensuring the avoidance of harmful changes,
- restoration – ensuring return to optimal levels of health once illness has occurred,
- amelioration – of illness and its effects.

Thus, it can be seen that the boundaries of community nursing are much wider and less distinct than those of the hospital nurse, and are often governed by diverse legal issues which encompass health related laws additional to nurse practice Acts. For this reason, it may not be so surprising that the notion of the community nurse as an agent of social control has gained precedence. However, as was seen in Chapter 5, both Dingwall and colleagues (1988) and Donzelot point out that the notion does not in anyway detract from the construct of community nursing as a caring profession, it merely means that community nursing care can help people to regulate their lives, and create relationships between the public and the state which are sensitive to public need (Figure 7.2).

The above considerations may make it easier to understand why it is that those concerned with the profession of community nursing such as politicians, managers and doctors have avoided consideration of the broad remit of community nursing care and the vast range of nursing responsibilities. By focusing only on the technical and procedural elements of the community nursing role, interested others may have found it only too easy to disguise from themselves the complexity of the interventions involved, and the fact that the range of caring interventions provided by community nurses required much more than a generic approach to care. On the contrary, as Nightingale herself recognised at the outset, the divergence of need in community settings requires a divergence in the focus of nursing care interventions that cannot be provided by a mere 'medical' focus of care.

To meet the current demand for both 'upstream' and 'downstream' foci of need and caring interventions, community nursing needs to clearly articulate what it means by care, and be able to identify the distinct contributions it can make to ensuring that social justice in health becomes a reality. Reverby (1987) observed that, although in the past nurses have been bound by a duty to care, they have been constrained to perform this duty in a society that on the whole has not valued caring. Thus, much of the caring work of community nurses, particularly perhaps those concerned with interventions of conservation, such as health visitors and school nurses has gone unnoticed. Only interventions that could be immediately noticed, such as those of district nurses and latterly the medically-orientated roles of practice nurses and nurse practitioners have been applauded. Thus, the invisibility of the complexity of care has, according to Radsma (1994), denigrated the work of some community nurses, and has made evaluation of their contribution difficult. The paucity of management technology has compounded this state of affairs by its ability only to measure procedure-orientated tasks, thereby disguising the 'price of care'. What then of the future? To meet the current need to ensure that health care is a requisite of social justice, the nursing profession itself, and the regulatory body in particular, need to be mindful of the fact that health is more than a means to an end, it is an end in itself. If community nursing wishes to construct itself as a caring profession, then the many faces of care required to achieve health and social wellbeing need to be recognised, and the divergence of constructs contained within the overarching term of 'community nurse' need to be made explicit.

Conclusion

The shifts towards new regimes in health and social care are driven by different but connected agendas. First, there is a growing concern over the efficacy of westernised medicine and increasing realisation that environmental and social determinants of health are more powerful resources than many technological medical interventions, and that prevention is much more cost effective than intervention (DoH 1998b). Second, there is the problem of escalating costs in the supply of hospital and medical care, and thirdly the culmination of growing concerns about the ethics and practice of institutionalisation of various groups within society such as the mentally ill, those with a learning disability, the elderly, children without parental support, and young offenders has led to a search for alternative care arrangements. These different agendas which underpin the 'regime of truth which is emerging in the twenty-first century appear then to contain ambivalent tensions which can be characterised by altruistic concerns to provide care, or pragmatic concerns to ensure control either of cost or of behaviour. The question pertinent to the construction of the image of community nursing is whether the profession subscribes to a caring or controlling role. It is increasingly recognised that the health of individuals and populations is affected by social determinants of health such as the environment, water quality, transport, housing, employment, education and training, crime and fear of crime and the access and availability of services. Public health therefore is not solely a health issue. In fact, the concept of public health medicine is a phenomenon dating only from the early 1990s (Macdonald 1998), when departments of community medicine or public health allied themselves to medicine (presumably for credibility and protection at a time when any kind of social rather than medical intervention in health was critically examined on grounds of economic expenditure (Symonds and Kelly 1998). Prior to this time, public health administration fluctuated between local authorities and health authorities in accordance with changes in government policy and strategy. Recent recognition of the importance of a broad range of health determinants appears to have re-awakened an interest in the importance of public health. The Secretary of State for Health stated in the House of Commons on 8 March 2001 that:

> Public health understood as the epidemiological analysis of the patterns and causes of population health and ill-health gets confused with 'public health' understood as health professionals trained in medicine . . . By a series of definitional sleights of hand the argument runs that the health of the population should mainly be improved by population-level health promotion and prevention which in turn is best delivered . . . or at least overseen and managed by medical consultants in public health.

Recent government health policy appears to have a health rather than an ill-ness focus and public health interventions are seen as key factors in making the UK a healthier nation. This shift towards the acceptance of a new 'regime' of truth is based on the definition of health as 'a resource for everyday life, not the object of living; it is a positive concept emphasising social and personal resources as well as physical capacities (WHO/EUR 1984).

Health is therefore seen as a social phenomenon, the province of groups and communities as well as individuals. According to Cowley (2000), this phenomenon has emerged from the science of 'salutogenesis' which is concerned with the identification of the factors which create health rather than disease, and with identifying factors that contribute to healing or to resistance to physiological or psychological breakdown.

Broadly then, public health can be seen as a caring strategy concerned with improving the health of populations and reducing health inequalities between social groups. It is based on the premise that the health of individuals is linked to the health of the population as a whole. Not only is the health of the poorest in society likely to be the worst, there is strong evidence pointing to the fact that, the greater the differential between the poor and the rich, the more likely it is that the health of the whole society is adversely affected (Appleby and Sayer 2001).

It would appear then that government are intent on introducing strategies based on a belief that improvement in health will ensure broader societal benefits, such as the social inclusion strategy:

> Social exclusion involves not only social but also economic and psychological isolation. Although people may know what affects their health, their hardship and isolation means that it is often more difficult for them to act on what they know. The best way to make a start on helping them to live healthier lives is to provide help and

support to enable them to participate in society and to help them improve their own economic and social circumstances. (DoH 1998)

The sentiments expressed in current policy appear to be widely divergent from primary care approaches which have been prevalent under previous governments. An editorial in the *Journal of Epidemiology and Community Health* (1995,**49**:113–16) clearly identifies the ideological differences between primary care and public health practice, which are illustrated in Table 7.2. Consideration of these tables clearly illustrates the significantly different foci of the respective approaches (see Table 7.1), and highlights the question of whether community nurses currently attached to primary care teams are likely to have any autonomy in decisions of whether their practice should be orientated towards a caring public health approach, or whether they are constrained to focus their interventions only on the controlling endeavours of the primary care team. Current public health challenges are to reduce premature deaths, improve health and reduce disease, act on environmental determinants of

Table 7.1   Some resources of public health and primary health care

Public health	Primary care
(a) Perspective	
• Care of populations	• Care of individual patients on practice list
• Environmental, social, organisational, and legislative interventions are of dominant importance	• 'Medical' interventions are of dominant importance
(b) Professional attitudes	
• Health requires organised efforts of society	• The consultation is the fundamental basis of health care
• Prevention is better than cure	• The care of the sick is the prime role, and prevention has a minor role
(c) Knowledge	
• Public health sciences (eg epidemiology/ medical statistics)	• Broad, clinical knowledge
• Organisational and management issues	• Local patterns of disease
• Policy-making	• Communication with individuals
• Administrative networks	• Personal circumstances of families/individuals
• Health status of large population/area	• Local community and its services
(d) Skills	
• Epidemiological and health services investigation/research	• Investigation and management of clinical problems
• Report and policy writing	• Consultation/communication
• Administration	• Small group leadership skills
• Communication with professional services	• Practice management
• Committee work	• Medical audit
	Nursing audit
(e) Information and material	
• Information on populations and their health in large areas	• The practice register and disease registers
• Access to health authority resources	• Information on individuals
• Access to non-medical staff, such as finance, computing, social care	• Access to local networks and primary care team

Table 7.2 The common agenda and illustration of the two approaches

Public health approach	Agenda	Primary care approach
• Serve whole population • Combination of methods including social and environmental policy change • Mass approaches to education • Educate educators and policy-makers • Seek expansion of funding base for prevention • Take responsibility for organisational aspects at a district/regional level	Improve health and prevent disease	• Serve patients on register/case-load • Focus on patients' illnesses and risk factors • Prevent by medical intervention • Lifestyle change by education • Undertake specific, but increasing range of activities in prevention
• Evaluation of the structure, process and outcome of services • Based primarily on epidemiological and demographic data, and on economic concepts	Effectiveness and efficiency of services	• Audit of clinical work and practice organisation • Based partly on subjective views of staff and patients
• Emphasis on needs of those who make no demand	Assessment of health needs	• Based mainly on demands of patients and contractual obligations
• Focus on disease causes; means of disease prevention, and on processes and outcomes of health care	Research	• Focus on management of common health problems, and on structures and processes of primary health care
• Develop local health policy and adapt and implement national and regional health policy	Policy-making and implementation	• Develop practice policy, and adopt and implement health authority policy

health address inequalities, promote social inclusion, facilitate and enable education training and employment, reduce teenage pregnancies, improve parenting, tackle drug use, safeguard and promote the rights of children and young people. Symonds and Kelly (1998) have shown that community nurses are ready to meet these challenges, provided that each of the professions included under the umbrella title 'community nurse' is allowed to contribute the full extent of their professional competence to the delivery of holistic care embraced by the spectrum of interventions which are contained between the opposite poles of care and cure.

In contrast to the recent developments in public health, concerns about community care still appear to focus on the fact that the main emphases of policy still appear to be directed towards those groups which are potentially destabilising forces in society (Symonds and Kelly 1998) such as older people, the mentally ill, children in need, carers, and minority groups and now, in addition, asylum seekers. In a paper commissioned by the United Council for Nurses Midwives and Health visitors, Warner and colleagues (1998) alert the Council to the challenge for nurses of the rapidly expanding elderly population, and the fact that by 2020 nearly half the population of the UK is likely to be over 45 years and that how within this population there will be increasing numbers of women, more mentally ill, increased numbers of people suffering from lifestyle disease such as overeating and obesity, increased numbers suffering from chronic con-communicable diseases and emergent and resurgent infectious diseases. Symonds and Kelly (1998) discuss how the discourses of community care have become 'codes' for the maintenance of social order of the groups identified above. The challenge to nurses who work with these groups is surely to carefully balance their interventions between care and control, adopting the definition of health quoted above (WHO/EUR 1984) and the fundamental tenets of the political ideology of patient Choice – well-informed consumers, empowerment and the loosening of professional control (Warner et al. 1998), in other words, to demonstrate how nursing interventions can foster the image of a civilising profession which is intent on reforming and redirecting the lives of people, as well as caring for them. Thereby, a convincing image of the value and worth of community nursing can surely be constructed.

Final conclusion

This book has attempted to unravel the complicated nature of the policy of health and community care and the profession of community nursing, and to show how it has been difficult for nurses to explain and establish the real nature of their roles because of the fact that others' notions of community nursing have been dominant. It has been shown how constructions of community nursing influenced by shifts towards the necessity for primary health care provision, and disillusionment with technological cures have been subjugated to the medical professions' desire for flexible and efficient services and, as a result, how professional discourses on the nature of care have been silenced. Thus it is concluded that the profession of community nursing has often found itself between a 'rock and a hard place' in trying to articulate the real nature of the care it provides.

Historically, it was shown that community nurses have been characterised as both carers and agents of social control, thus the nature of their work may have been conceptually confused. Literature shows that there is a great deal of obfuscation surrounding the concept of care and that many aspects of the concept are intangible, couched in linguistic ambivalences and overwhelmed by gender and political considerations. Thus, according to Dingwall and colleagues (1988), if community nurses wish to articulate their role and function they should be able to determine that their role is a pragmatic way of responding to the problems of particular groups so that they can maintain sufficient order to plan and control their lives. This suggests that community nurses should value a regulatory function and be able to demonstrate that the exercise of social control through health care can provide a positive experience for populations in the community. This does not mean that community nurse roles should be dictatorial or controlling, merely that they are capable of providing social support and education for certain population groups. However, the ambivalent tensions experienced by community nurses often means that their practice is more focused on interventions of a curing nature. The value placed on the latter appears to have been to the detriment of the former, a situation which has been even more confused by the fact that latterly a prevalent belief in a unified profession of community nurses (Hyde 1995) has confused the issue of the real nature of community nursing even more. This development has hidden the fact that the preferred focus of the various branches of community nursing may vary according to different concepts of practice. Interventions over a wide range of social and health care result in different foci of care and a range of different practice from promotion, prevention, intervention and palliative care. Each type of intervention is as important as the other, and consequently all must be valued. However, efforts to control spending in health care, a disregard for the value of preventive care, and a reluctance to recognise that the primary cause of ill health was poverty, have led to a disregard of the type of community nursing interventions required to meet the demands for public health. This has been a development that has disenfranchised some branches of community nursing and ignored the different nature of the caring interventions they could offer.

More recently the realisation of the value of public health intervention and the policy discourses of equity, responsible parenting, work and social inclusion have recognised the need for nursing interventions that through the process of social control can provide a regulatory and supportive service for excluded groups. Whereas in the past an emphasis on a disease model of health may have made public health interventions of a socio-economic nature redundant, a modern interest in the importance of public health has brought about a revival in the need for public health workers able to work in multidisciplinary settings, who are conscious of the 'joined-up' nature of health and social deprivation. However, this notion has been slow to be adopted by the profession of community nursing, despite the fact that government policy is peppered with the rhetoric of public health. The reliance of the majority community nurses on a medical model of care to provide a framework for the interpretation of new policy appears to have led the profession of community nursing into a 'blind alley' where it is increasingly responsible for 'low-tech' care. This outcome has been seen by many as disadvantaging community nurses, such as school nurses and health visitors who are concerned with the necessity for public health services.

Recent policy has challenged community nurses to examine the part that they play in the delivery of the 'New Public Health'. Although many recognise that preventive social care should be given priority, it has been quite difficult for community nurses themselves to articulate the exact nature of their role in meeting such demands. This in part may have been due to the pressures placed on all community nurses to conform to re-active models of caring intervention, but it may also have been due to a poor conceptual understanding of the different aspects of caring and the diversity of the roles required to provide comprehensive and adequate services to protect public health.

Finally, it was shown how the current direction of policy, aimed at the social inclusion of vulnerable groups has challenged all branches of community nursing to distinguish the exact nature of various roles. It was seen that, despite adverse influences of managerialism and medical orientations of care, community nurses are beginning to articulate and demonstrate the diverse nature of their roles thereby giving the public and other professions the opportunity to value the diversity of the profession of community nursing.

Bibliography

Abel-Smith, B. (1960). *History of Nursing*. London: Heinemann.

Abel-Smith, B. (1964). *The Hospitals 1800–1948: A Study in Social Administration in England and Wales*. London: Heinemann.

Ackroyd, S. (1998). 'Nurses.' In Laffin, M. (ed.), *Beyond Bureaucracy*. London: Avebury.

Aggleton, P. (1990). *Health*. London: Routledge.

Alderman, H. (2000). 'The Bradford Experience.' *Primary Health Care*, **101**, 8 February.

Allsop, J. (1984). *Health Policy and the National Health Service*. London: Longman.

Altman, D. (1986). *AIDS and the New Puritanism*. London: Pluto Press.

Appleby, F. and Sayer, L. (2001). 'Public Health Nursing – Health Visiting.' In Sines, D., Appleby, F. and Raymond, E. (eds), *Community Healthcare Nursing*. Oxford: Blackwell Scientific.

Armstrong, D. (1983). *Political Anatomy of the Body: Medical Knowledge in Britain in the Twentieth Century*. Cambridge: Cambridge University Press.

Armstrong, D. (1986). 'The Invention of Infant Morality.' *Sociology of Health and Illness*, **8**, 211–32.

Armstrong, D. (1993). 'Public Health Spaces and the Fabrication of Identity.' *Sociology*, **27**: 3, 393–410.

Armstrong, D. (1995). 'The Rise of Surveillance Medicine.' *Sociology of Health and Illness*, **17**: 3, 393–404.

Ashton, J. and Seymour, H. (1988). *The New Public Health*. Buckingham: Open University.

Attfield, J. (1989). 'Inside Pram Town: A Case Study of Harlow 1951–1961.' In Attfield, J. and Kirkham, P. (eds), *A View From the Interior: Feminism, Women and Design*. London: The Women's Press.

Attfield, J. and Kirkham, P. (eds) (1989). *A View from the Interior: Feminism, Women and Design*. London: The Women's Press

Audit Commission for Local Authorities in England and Wales (1994). *Seen But Not Heard: Co-ordinating Community Child Health and Social Services for Children in Need*. London: HMSO.

Audit Commission (1999). *First Assessment: A Review of District Nursing Services in England and Wales*. London: AC.

Aurora, S. and Irvine, S. (2000). 'Developing Health Improvement Programmes.' *Journal of Interprofessional Care*, **141**, 9–18.

Baggot, R. (2000). *Public Health, Policy and Politics*. Basingstoke: Macmillan Press – now Palgrave Macmillan.

Baly, M. E. (1973). *Nursing and Social Change*. London: Routledge.

Baly, M. (1986). *Florence Nightingale and the Nursing Legacy*. London: Croom Helm.

Baly, M. E. (1987). *District Nursing* (2nd edn). Guildford: Biddles.

Baly, M. E. (1987a). *A History of the Queens Institute*. London: Croom Helm.

Bamford, T. (1990). *The Future of Social Work*. Basingstoke: Macmillan Press – now Palgrave Macmillan.

Banerji, D. (1984). *Primary Health Care: Selective or Comprehensive.* World Health Forum, vol. 5.

Bartlett, W. (1991). 'Quasi Markets and Contracts: A Markets and Hierarchies Perspective on the NHS Reforms.' *Public Money and Management,* 11, 53–61.

Bartlett, W. and Le Grand, J. (1993). *Quasi Markets and Social Policy.* Basingstoke: Macmillan – now Palgrave Macmillan.

Bartley, M., Blane, D. and Davey Smith, G. (1998). *The Sociology of Health Inequalities.* Oxford: Blackwell.

Baum, F. and Sanders, D. (1995). 'Can Health Promotion and Primary Health Care Achieve Health for All without a Return to a More Radical Agenda?' *Health Promotion International,* 10: 2, 149–60.

Baumgart, A. (1998). *Called to Account – Nursing Education for Yesterday or Tomorrow.* Proceedings of the Olive Anstey International Nursing Conference, Perth.

Bearshaw, V. and Robinson, K. (1990). *New for Old? Prospects for Nursing in the 1990s.* Research Report No. 8. London: King's Fund Institute.

Beattie, A. (1993). 'The Changing Boundaries of Health.' In Beattie, A., Gott, M., Jones, L. and Sidell, M. (eds), *Health and Well-being.* Basingstoke: Macmillan – now Palgrave Macmillan.

Benzeval, M., Judge, K. and Whitehead, M. (1995). *Tackling Inequalities in Health.* London: King's Fund.

Beveridge, W. (1942). *Social Insurance and Allied Services.* Cmnd 6404, London: HMSO.

Birch, H. (2001). 'The Extended Role of the Nurse – Opportunity or Threat?' *Human Fertility.* Cambridge, 43, 138–44.

Blaxter, M. (1990). *Health and Lifestyles.* London: Routledge.

Bond, S., Rhodes, T., Philips, P., Setters, J., Foy, C. and Bond, J. (1990). 'HIV Infection and AIDS in England: The Experience, Knowledge and Intentions of Community Nursing Staff.' *Journal of Advanced Nursing,* 15, 249–55.

Booth, C. (1902). *Life and Labour of the People of London.* London: Macmillan

Bourke, J. (1996). *Dismembering the Male: Men's Bodies, Britain and the Great War.* London: Reaktion Books.

Bowlby, J. (1953). *Care and the Growth of Love.* New York: Basic Books.

Boyd Orr, J. (1936). *Food, Health and Income.* London: Macmillan – now Palgrave Macmillan.

British Medical Journal (1999). 'UK Community Groups Reject Mental Health Reforms.' *BMJ,* 27 November, 7222, 1389.

Bunker, J., Frazier, H. and Mostelle, F. (1994). 'Improving Health: Measuring Effects of Medical Care.' *Millbank Quarterly,* 72, 2.

Burnett, J. (1982). *Destiny Obscure.* Harmondsworth: Penguin Books.

Burnett, J. (1986). *A Social History of Housing 1815–1985.* London: Routledge.

Butterworth, T. (1988). 'Breaking the Boundaries.' *Nursing Times,* 84, 47.

Bynum, W. (1994). *Science and the Practice of Medicine in the Nineteenth Century.* Cambridge: Cambridge University Press.

Bytheway, B. and Johnson, J. (1998). 'The Social Construction of "Carers".' In Symonds, A. and Kelly, A. (eds), *The Social Construction of Community Care.* Basingstoke: Macmillan Press – now Palgrave Macmillan.

Cabinet Office (1999). *Modernising Government.* London: HMSO.

Campbell, B. (1988). *Unofficial Secrets; Child Sexual Abuse and the Cleveland Case.* London: Virago.

Carpenito, L. J. (1993). *Nursing Diagnosis: Application to Clinical Practice* (5th edn), Philadelphia: J. B. Lippincott.

Carpenter, M. (1980). 'Asylum Nursing before 1914: A Chapter in the History of Labour.' Davies, C. (ed.), *Re-writing Nursing History.* London: Croom Helm.

Charley, I. (1954). *The Birth of Industrial Nursing*. London: Bailliere Tindall.

Chell, S. (2000). 'Men's Health: Slugs and Snails.' *Practice Nursing*, **11**: 17, 6–9. December.

Chen, C. H., Wang, S. Y. and Chang, M. Y. (2001). 'Women's Perceptions of Helpful and Unhelpful Nursing Behaviours during Labour.' *Birth*, September, **283**, 180–5.

Chen, S. (1999). *Citizens and Taxes*. Fabian Pamphlet 593, London: Fabian Society.

Churchill, D., Allen, J., Pringle, M., Hippisley-Cox, J., Ebdon, D., Macpherson, M. and Bradley, S. (2000). 'Consultation Patterns and Provision of Contraception in General Practice before Teenage Pregnancy: Case-control Study.' *British Medical Journal*, **321**, 486–9.

Clark, J. (2000). 'Old Wine in New Bottles: Delivering Nursing in the 21st Century.' *Journal of Nursing Scholarship*, 2000, **32**: 1, 11–15, Sigma Theta Tau International.

Clark, J., Buttigieg, M., Bodycombe-James, M., Eaton, N., Kelly, A., Merrell, J., Palmer-Thomas, J., Parke, S. and Symonds, A. (2000). *Recognising the Potential: The Review of Health Visiting and School Health Services in Wales*. University of Wales Swansea.

Clay, T. (1998). 'Community Service Left to Struggle.' *Nursing Times*, **84**: 6, 6.

Clendon, J. and White, G. (2001). 'The Feasibility of a Nurse-practitioner-led Primary Health Care Clinic in a School Setting: A Community Needs Analysis.' *The Journal of Advanced Nursing*, **34**: 2, 171–8. April.

Cochrane, A. (1971). *Effectiveness and Efficiency: Random Reflections on Health Services*. London: Nuffield Provincial Hospital Trusts.

Cole and Furbey (1994). *The Eclipse of Council Housing*. London: Routledge.

Colliere, M. (1986). 'Invisible Care and Invisible Women as Health Care Providers.' *International Journal of Nursing Studies*, **23**, 95–112.

Community Practitioner (1999). 'Sure Start Doubts Remain.' *Community Practitioner*, **72**: 5, 111.

Community Practitioners' and Health Visitors' Association (1997). *Making the Difference: Demonstrating the Effectiveness of Health Visiting*. London: CPHVA.

Community Practitioners' and Health Visitors' Association (2000). Response to the Green Paper on Housing – 'Quality and Choice: A Decent Home for All.' http://www.msfcphva.org/members/net

Coulton, M., Drury, C. and Williams, M. (1998). 'Working with Children in Need under the Children Act 1989.' In Symonds, A. and Kelly, A. (eds), *The Social Construction of Community Care*. Basingstoke: Macmillan Press – now Palgrave Macmillan.

Council Education and Training of Health Visitors (CETHV) (1977). *An Investigation into the Principles of Health Visiting*. London: Whitefriars Press.

Cowley, S. (2000). 'Situation and Process in Health Visiting.' In Appelton, J. and Cowley, S. (eds), *The Search for Health Needs: Research for Health Visiting Practice*. Basingstoke: Macmillan Press – now Palgrave Macmillan.

Crossick, J. (1978). *An Artisan Elite in Victorian Society*. London: Croom Helm.

Cumming, E. and J. (1957). *Closed Ranks: An Experiment in Mental Health Education*. Boston: Harvard University Press.

Dahlgren, G. (1996). 'The Need for Intersectional Action for Health.' In European Health Policy Conference: *Opportunities for the Future, Vol. 2, Intersectional Action for Health*. Copenhagen: WHO Regional Office for Europe.

Dalley, G. (1988). *Ideologies of Caring: Rethinking Community and Collectivism*. Basingstoke: Macmillan – now Palgrave Macmillan.

Daniel, K. (2000). 'Brilliantly Tackled.' *Community Practitioner*, **73**: 8, 708–9. August.

Davies, C. (1988). 'The Health Visitor as Mother's Friend.' *Social History of Medicine*, **1**, 1, 39–59.

Davies, C. (1995). *Gender and the Professional Predicament in Nursing.* Buckingham: Open University Press.

Davin, A. (1978). 'Imperialism and Motherhood.' *History Workshop*, **5**, 9–65.

Davin, A. (1996). *Growing Up Poor: Home, School and Street in London 1870–1914.* London: Rivers Oram.

Davison, D., Davey-Smith, G. and Frankel, S. (1991). 'Lay Epidemiology and the Prevention Paradox: The Implications of Coronary Candidacy for Health Education.' *Sociology of Health and Illness*, **13**: 1, 1–19.

Daykin, N. and Naidoo, J. (1995). 'Feminist Critiques of Health Promotion.' In Bunton, R., Nettleton, S. and Burrows, R. (eds), *The Sociology of Health Promotion.* London: Routledge.

Dean, H. (1999). 'Introduction.' In Ellis, K. and Dean, H. (eds), *Social Policy and the Body: Transitions in Corporeal Discourse.* New York: Macmillan.

Dean, M. and Bolton, G. (1980). 'The Administration of Poverty and the Development of Nursing Practice in 19th Century England.' In Davies, C. (ed.), *Re-Writing Nursing History.* London: Croom Helm.

Dennis, N and Erdos, G. (1993). *Families Without Fatherhood.* London: Institute of Economic Affairs.

Department for Education and Employment (2000). *Connexions; The Best Start in Life for Every Young Person.* London: DfEE.

Department for Education and Employment (1999). *Design of the New Deal for 18–24 Year Olds.* London: DfEE.

Department of Health (1979). *Nursing Midwifery and Health Visiting Act.* London: HMSO.

Department of Health (1980). *Inequalities in Health (Black Report).* London: HMSO.

Department of Health (1989). *Working for Patients.* London: HMSO.

Department of Health (1989a). *Caring for People, Community Care in the Next Decade and Beyond.* London: HMSO.

Department of Health (1989b). *General Practice in the National Health Service: The 1990 Contract.* London: HMSO.

Department of Health (1991). *The Patient's Charter.* London: HMSO.

Department of Health (1991). *The Health of the Nation.* Cmnd 523. London: HMSO.

Department of Health (1992). *The Health of the Nation: A Strategy for Health in England.* London: HMSO.

Department of Health (1993). *A Strategy for Nursing, Midwifery and Health Visiting.* London: HMSO.

Department of Health (1997). *The New NHS, Modern Dependable.* Cmnd 3807. London: HMSO.

Department of Health (1998). *The New NHS Modern and Dependable: A National Framework for Assessing Performance.* London: The Stationery Office.

Department of Health (1998a). *Our Healthier Nation.* London: HMSO.

Department of Health (1998b). *Independent Inquiry into Inequalities of Health (Acheson Report).* London: HMSO.

Department of Health (1998c). *NHS Priorities and Planning Guidance.* London: HMSO.

Department of Health (1999). *Modernising Mental Health Services.* London: HMSO.

Department of Health (2000). *The NHS Plan: A Plan for Investment, A Plan for Reform.* Cmnd 4818-1. London: The Stationery Office.

Department of Health (2000a). *A Health Service of all the Talents; Developing the NHS Workforce* – Consultation Document on the review of workforce planning. London: The Stationery Office.

Department of Health (2002). *Delivering the NHS Plan.* London: HMSO.

Department of Health (2002a). *Tackling Health Inequalities: The Results of a Consultation Exercise.* London: HMSO.

DHSS (1976). *Prevention and Health: Everybody's Business.* London: HMSO.

DHSS (1979–81). *Development Team for the Mentally Handicapped.* Reports. London: DHSS.

DHSS (1980). *Organisational and Management Problems of Mental Illness Hospitals.* Report of a working group. London: DHSS.

DHSS (1980a). Working Group on Inequalities in Health (Chair: Sir D. Black) (The Black Report). London: HMSO.

DHSS (1983). *NHS Management Inquiry* (Griffiths Report). London: HMSO.

DHSS (1986). *Neighbourhood Nursing – A Focus for Care.* Report of the Community Nursing Review. Cumberlege Report, London: HMSO.

DHSS (1988). *Community Care: An Agenda for Action.* The Griffiths Community Care Report. London: HMSO.

DHSS (1987). *Promoting Better Health: The Government's Programme for Improving Primary Health Care.* London: HMSO.

DHSS (1990). *The NHS and Community Care Act.* London: HMSO.

Department of Social Security (1998). *Proportion of Children and the Population in Households below 50% of Average Income 1976–1996 UK.* London: HMSO.

Department of Social Security (1999). *Opportunity for All: Tackling Poverty and Social Exclusion.* Cmnd 4445. London: HMSO.

Department of Transport and Environment (1997). *Involving Communities in Urban and Rural Regeneration.* London: HMSO.

Dingwall, R. (1974). 'A Team Role for Ancilliary Staff.' *Health and Social Services Journal,* September 7, 2032–33.

Dingwall, R. (1975). 'Health Visitors and Social Workers – Where are the Boundaries?' *Health and Social Service Journal,* November 22, 2608–9.

Dingwall, R. (1977). 'Collectivism, Regionalism and Feminism: Health Visiting and British Social Policy 1850–1975.' *Journal of Social Policy,* **6**, 291–315.

Dingwall, R. (1982). 'Community Nursing and Civil Liberty.' *Journal of Advanced Nursing,* **7**, 337–46.

Dingwall, R., Rafferty, A. and Webster, C. (1988). *An Introduction to the Social History of Nursing.* London: Routledge.

Digby, A. (1985). *Madness, Morality and Medicine.* Cambridge: Cambridge University Press.

Dolan, J. (1973). *Nursing in Society – A Historical Perspective.* London: Saunders.

Donnison, J. (1977) *Midwives and Medical Men.* London: Heinemann.

Donzelot, J. (1980). *The Policing of Families.* London: Hutchinson.

Drake, R. (1998). 'Professionals and the Voluntary Sector.' In Symonds, A. and Kelly, A., (eds), *The Social Construction of Community Care.* Basingstoke: Macmillan Press – now Palgrave Macmillan.

Drakeford, M. and Butler, I. (2000). *Scandal and Social Policy.* Basingstoke: Macmillan Press – now Palgrave Macmillan.

Driver, S. and Martell, L. (1997). 'New Labour's Communitarianisms.' *Critical Social Policy,* **17**: 3, 27–44.

Dunlop, M. J. (1986). 'Is a Science of Caring Possible?' *Journal of Advanced Nursing,* **11**, 661–70.

Dwork, D. (1986). *War is Good for Babies and Other Young Children: A History of the Infant and Child Welfare Movement in England 1898–1918.* London: Tavistock.

Dyhouse, C. (1978). 'Working Class Mothers and Infant Mortality in England 1895–1914.' *Journal of Social History,* **12**, 248–68.

Editorial (1995). 'Public Health Medicine and Primary Health Care: Convergent, Divergent, or Parallel Paths?' *Journal of Epidemiology and Community Health,* **49**, 113–16.

Ehrenreich, B. and English, D. (1979). *For Her own Good: 150 years of the Experts' Advice to Women.* London: Virago.

Ellis, K. (2000). 'Welfare and Bodily Order.' In Ellis, K. and Dean, H. (eds), *Social Policy and the Body.* Basingstoke: Macmillan Press – now Palgrave Macmillan.

Enthoven, A. (1985). *Reflections on Management of the NHS.* Oxford: Nuffield Hospital Trust.

Etzioni, A. (1995). *The Spirit of Community.* London: Fontana.

European Conference on Nursing (1988). Conference Report, *Journal of Advanced Nursing, 1989,* **14**, 599–602.

Farrington, D. (1995). 'Intensive Health Visiting and the Prevention of Juvenile Crime.' *Health Visitor,* **68**: 3, 100–2.

Fatchett, A. (1990). 'Health Visiting: A Withering Profession?' *Journal of Advanced Nursing,* **15**, 215–22.

Fatchett, A. (1994). *Politics, Policy and Nursing.* London: Balliere and Tindall.

Finch, J. and Groves, D. (1983). *A Labour of Love: Women, Work and Caring.* London: Routledge and Kegan Paul.

Florin and Rosen (1999). 'Evaluating NHS Direct – Early Findings Raise Questions about Expanding the Service.' *British Medical Journal,* **319**: 7201, 5–6.

Flynn, R. (1988). 'Political Acquiescence, Privatisation and Residualisation in British Housing Policy.' *Journal of Social Policy,* **17**: 3, 289–312.

Forrest, R. and Murie, A. (1988). *Selling the Welfare State.* London: Routledge.

Foster, J. (1974). *Class Struggle and the Industrial Revolution.* London: Methuen.

Foucault, M. (1973). *Birth of the Clinic.* London: Tavistock.

Foucault, M. (1974). *Archaeology of Knowledge.* London: Tavistock.

Foucault, M. (1980). *Power and Knowledge.* Brighton: Harvester Press.

Foucault, M. (1991). 'Governmentality.' In Burchell, G., Gordon, C. and Miller, P. (eds), *The Foucault Effect.* Brighton: Harvester Wheatsheaf.

Fox, E. (1993). 'An Honourable Calling or a Despised Occupation: Licensed Midwifery and its Relationship to District Nursing in England and Wales before 1948.' *Society for Social History of Medicine,* **6**: 2, 237–59.

Fox, N. (1997). 'Is There Life after Foucault?' In Petersen, A. and Bunton, R. (eds), *Foucault Health and Medicine.* London: Routledge.

Frost, H. and Stein, M. (1989). *The Politics of Child Welfare.* Herts: Harvester Wheatsheaf.

Gale, C. and Martyn, C. (1995). 'Dummies and the Health of Hertfordshire Infants 1911–1939.' *Society for Social History of Medicine,* 231–55.

Garmarnikow, E. (1978). 'Sexual Division of Labour: The Case of Nursing.' In Kuhn, A. and Wolpe, A. M. (eds), *Feminism and Materialism: Women and Modes of Production.* London: Routledge and Kegan Paul.

Gaudie, E. (1974). *Cruel Habitations.* London: Unwin University Books.

Giddens, A. (1994). *Beyond Left and Right: The New Radicalism.* London: Polity Press.

Giddens, A. (1998). 'After the Left's Paralysis.' *New Statesman,* May 1, 18–21.

Gillespie, R. (1997). 'Managers and Professionals.' In North and Bradshaw (eds), *Perspectives in Health Care.* Basingstoke: Macmillan – now Palgrave Macmillan.

Gloyne, S. R. (1944). *Social Aspects of Tuberculosis.* London: Faber and Faber.

Goldthorpe, D. and Lockwood, D. (1969). *The Affluent Worker in the Class Structure.* Cambridge: Cambridge University Press.

Goodwin, S. (1988). 'Whither Health Visiting?' *Health Visitor,* **61**, 379–83.

Gordon, L. (1989). *Heroes of Their Own Lives.* London: Virago.

Gournay, K. (1994). 'Redirecting the Emphasis to Serious Mental Illness.' *Nursing Times,* **90**: 25, 40–1.

Griffiths, J. (2001). 'Meeting Personal Hygiene Needs in the Community; A District Nursing Perspective on the Health and Social Care Divide.' *Health and Social Care in the Community,* 1998, July, **64**, 234–40.

Harriott, S. and Matthews, L. (1998). *Social Housing.* London: Longman.

Harrison, S. and Pollitt, C. (1994). *Controlling the Professionals.* Buckingham: Open University.

Health Committee Report (1992). Session 1991–1992 [Chairman: Mr Nicholas Winterton] *Maternity Services*, vol. 1. London: HMSO.

Heginbotham, C. and Bosanquet, N. (1995). 'A Promise of Better Things to Come.' *Health Service Journal*, 27 July, 26–7.

Hennessy, D. (1995). 'A Changing Health Service Requires a Changing Workforce.' In Littlewood, J. (ed.), *Current Issues in Community Nursing*. London: Churchill Livingstone.

H M Prison Service (HMPS) (1997). HMI *Thematic Inspection of Young Prisoners*. London: HMPS.

HMSO (1972). *Report of the Committee on Nursing* [Chairman: Lord Briggs]. Cmnd 5115. London: HMSO.

HMSO (1999). *With Respect to Old Age. Report of the Royal Commission on Long Term Care* (Chair: Sir Stewart Sutherland). London: HMSO.

Hobcraft, J. (1998). *Intergenerational and Life Course Transmission of Social Exclusion: Influences of Childhood Poverty, Family Disruption and Contact with the Police*. Case Paper 15. London: London School of Economics.

Hobsbawm, E. (1968). *Labouring Men*. London: Weidenfeld and Nicholson.

Hogrefe, P. (1975). *Tudor Women, Commoners and Queens*. Ames, Iowa: Iowa State University.

Holliday, M. and Parker, D. (1997). 'Florence Nightingale, Feminism and Nursing.' *Journal of Advanced Nursing*, **26**, 483–8.

Homans, H. and Aggleton, P. (1988). 'Health Education, HIV Infection and AIDS.' In Aggleton and Homans (eds), *Social Aspects of AIDS*. Lewes: Falmer Press.

Home Office (1998). *Supporting Families: A Consultation Document*: London: The Stationery Office.

Hunt, S. and Symonds, A. (1995). *The Social Meaning of Midwifery*. London: Macmillan – now Palgrave Macmillan.

Husserl, E. (1931). *Ideas* [W. R. Boyce Gibson, Trans.] London: George Allen and Unwin.

Hutt, A. (1933). *The Condition of the Working Class in Britain*. London: Gollancz.

Hyde, V. (1995). 'Community Nursing: A Unified Discipline?' In Cain, P., Hyde, V. and Howkins, E. (eds), *Community Nursing*. London: Arnold.

Independent (1996). 'Vulnerable Young Are Forced Out of Their Homes.' April 17, 7.

Independent (1999). 26 November, Review, 1.

Johnson, N. (1999). 'The Personal Social Services and Community Care.' In Powell, M. (ed.), *New Labour, New Welfare State?* London: Policy Press.

Jones, A. M. (2000). *Do Social Care Needs Influence the Nature of District Nursing Provision?: A Survey of District Nursing Services in an NHS Trust*. (Unpublished Master's Thesis), University of Wales Swansea.

Jones, H. (1994). *Health and Society in Twentieth Century Britain*. London: Longman.

Jones, S. (2000). *The Incidence of Verbal Abuse which District Nurses Accept as an Inevitable Consequence of Patient Care*. (Unpublished Master's Thesis), University of Wales Swansea.

Joseph, J. and Sumption, J. (1979). *Equality*. London: John Murray.

Joseph Rowntree Foundation (1998). *Poverty and Exclusion in Rural Britain: The Dynamics of Low Income and Employment*. York: Joseph Rowntree Foundation Findings 418.

Keating, P. (1976). *Into Unknown England*. Manchester: Manchester University Press.

Kelly, A. (1998). 'Professionals and the Changed Environment.' In Symonds, A. and Kelly, A. (eds), *The Social Construction of Community Care*. Basingstoke: Macmillan Press – now Palgrave Macmillan.

Kelly, A., Mabbett, G. and Thome, R. (1998). 'Professions and Community Nursing.' In Symonds, A. and Kelly, A. (eds), *The Social Construction of Community Care*. Basingstoke: Macmillan Press – now Palgrave Macmillan.

Klainberg, M., Holzemer, S., Leonard M. and Arnold, J. (1998). *Community Health Nursing. An Alliance for Health*. New York: McGraw Hill.

Klein, R. (1974). *The Politics of the NHS*. London: Longman.

Klein, R (1989). *The Politics of the NHS*. London: Longman.

Kurtz, R. J. and Wang, J. (1991). 'The Caring Ethic: More than Kindness, The Core of Nursing Science.' *Nursing Forum*, **26**: 1, 4–8.

Land, H. (1999). 'New Labour, New Families?' *Social Policy Review*, **11**, 127–44.

Lashmar, P. (2000). *Dagenham My Dagenham*. The Independent Review, 25 April, 1.

Leap, N. and Hunter, B. (1993). *The Midwife's Tale*. London: Scarlett Press.

Le Fanu, J. (1986). 'Diet and Disease – Nonsense and Non-science.' In Anderson, D. (ed.), *A Diet of Reason*. London: Social Affairs Unit.

Leat, D. (1995). 'Funding Matters.' In Davis Smith, J., Rochester, C. and Hedley, R. (eds), *An Introduction to the Voluntary Sector*. London: Routledge.

Leather, S. (1996). *The Making of Modern Malnutrition: An Overview of Food Poverty in the UK*. London: Caroline Walker Trust.

Le Grand, J. (1998). 'The Third Way Begins with CORA.' *New Statesman*, 6 March, 26–7.

Leipert, B. D. (2001). 'Feminism and Public Health Nursing: Partners for Health.' *School Inq. Nursing Practice*, Spring; **15**: 1, 49–61.

Lewis, J. (1980). *Politics of Motherhood; Child and Maternal Welfare in England 1900–1939*. London: Croom Helm.

Lewis, J. (1986). *What Price Community Medicine?* Brighton: Harvester Wheatsheaf.

Lewis, J. (2000). *A Study of Health Visitors' Perceptions of Public Health Practice*. (Unpublished Master's Thesis), University of Wales Swansea.

Lindsey, E. and Harrick, G. (1996). 'Health Promoting Nursing Practice: The Demise of the Nursing Process.' *Journal of Advanced Nursing*, **2**: 3, 106–12.

Lister, R. (1999). 'New Welfare: An Analysis of the Government's Approach.' *Community Practitioner*, **72**: 2, 20–2.

Littlewood, J. (ed.) (1995). *Current Issues in Community Nursing*. London: Churchill Livingstone.

Llewellyn, S. and Trent, D. (1987). *Nursing in the Community. Psychology in Action*. British Psychological Society.

Loane, M. (1909). *Englishman's Castle*. London: Edward Arnold.

Lund, B. (1996). *Housing Problems and Housing Policy*. London: Longman.

Lyne, P. A. (1997). *Taskforce for Continuing Education and Practice: The Future of Nurses, Midwives and Health Visitors*. Cardiff: Nursing Research Centre School of Nursing Studies.

Macdonald, J. (1998). *Primary Health Care, Medicine in its Place*. London: Earthscan Publications.

Mackenzie, N. and J. (1979). *The First Fabians*. Guildford: Quartet Books.

Mackintosh, C. (1997). 'A Historical Study of Men in Nursing.' *Journal of Advanced Nursing*, **26**, 232–6.

Macleod Clark, J. (1993). *From Sick Nursing to Health Nursing: Evolution or Revolution?* London: Wilson Barnett.

Mann, K. (1992). *The Making of an English 'Underclass'?* Milton Keynes: Open University Press.

Marshall, T. (1950). *Citizenship and Social Class*. Cambridge: Cambridge University Press.

Marwick, A. (1974). *War and Social Change in the Twentieth Century*. Basingstoke: Macmillan – now Palgrave Macmillan.

Mayall, B. (1996). *Children, Health and the Social Order*. Buckingham: OUP.

McCarthy (ed.) (1989). *The New Politics of Welfare: An Agenda for the 1990s*. London: Macmillan – now Palgrave Macmillan.

McClelland, A. (1996). 'Working Girls and Working Women.' *Health Visitor Journal*, **69**: 7, 265–8.

McEwan, M. (1951). *Health Visiting*. London: Faber and Faber.

McGonigle, G. and Kirby, J. (1936). *Poverty and Public Health*. London: Gollancz.

McKeigue, P. (1991). 'Patterns of Health and Disease in the Elderly of Minority Ethnic Groups.' In Squires, A. (ed.), *Multicultural Healthcare and Rehabilitation*. London: Edward Arnold.

McKeown, T. (1976). *The Role of Medicine: Dream, Mirage or Nemesis?* London: Nuffield Provincial Hospital Trust.

McKie, E. (1963). *Venture in Faith*. Liverpool: Liverpool and District Family Service Unit.

McKinley, J. B. and Arches, J. (1985). 'Towards the Proletarianisation of Physicians.' *International Journal of Health Services* **5**: 2, 161–95.

McMurray, A. (1990). *Community Health Nursing*. London: Churchill Livingstone.

McQueen, D. (1988). 'Thoughts on the Ideological Origins of Health Promotion.' *Health Promotion*, **4**: 4, 339–42.

Means, R. and Smith, R. (1994). *Community Care, Policy and Practice*. Basingstoke: Macmillan – now Palgrave Macmillan.

Ministry of Health (MOH) (1937). *Report on Maternal Mortality*. Cmnd 5422, London: HMSO.

Ministry of Health, Department of Health for Scotland, and Ministry of Labour and National Service (1947). *Report of the Working Party on the Recruitment and Training of Nurses* (Chairman: Sir Robert Wood). London: HMSO.

Ministry of Health (1956). *Report of the Committee of Enquiry into the Cost of the NHS* (Guillebaud Report). Cmnd 9663. London: HMSO.

Ministry of Health (1956a). *An Inquiry into Health Visiting* (Jameson Report). London: HMSO.

Ministry of Housing (1961). *Homes for Today and Tomorrow (The Parker Morris Report)*. London: HMSO.

Mitchell, M. (1999). 'Disciplinary Intentions and Resistances Around "Safer Sex".' In Ellis, K. and Dean, H. (eds), *Social Policy and the Body*. Basingstoke: Macmillan Press – now Palgrave Macmillan.

Moon, G. (1997). 'Markets and Choice.' North, P. and Bradshaw, J. (eds), *Perspectives in Health Care*. Basingstoke: Macmillan – now Palgrave Macmillan.

Mooney, G. (1997). Unpublished Master's thesis, University of Wales Swansea.

Mooney, G. and Symonds, A. (2001). ' "They said just come in for the day": Patients' Experience of Day Care Surgery." *Primary Health Care Research and Development* **2**, 55–61.

Morris, L. (1994). *Dangerous Classes*. London: Routledge.

Morrow, H. (1988). 'Nurses, Nursing and Women.' *International Nursing Review*, **35**: 1, 22–5.

Moylan, S., Millar, J. and Davies, R. (1984). *For Richer For Poorer?: A Department of Health and Social Security Cohort Study of Unemployed Men*. London: HMSO.

Murray, C. (1990). *The Emerging British Underclass*. London: Institute of Economic Affairs.

Murray, C. (1994). *Underclass: The Crisis Deepens*. London: London Institute of Economic Affairs.

National Assembly for Wales (NAfW) (2000). *Promoting Health and Well-being; A Consultation Document*. Cardiff: NafW.

National Assembly for Wales (NAfW) (2001). *Improving Health in Wales: A Plan for the NHS with its Partners*. Cardiff: NafW.

National Assembly for Wales (NAfW) (2001a). *Promoting Health and Well Being: Implementing the National Health Promotion Strategy*. Cardiff: NafW.

National Association for the Care and Resettlement of Offenders (NACRO) (1999). *Youth Offending and Health: The Role of YOTs.* London: NACRO Briefing.

National Health Service Management Executive (1992). *Extension of the Hospital and Community Health Services: Elements of the GP Fundholding Scheme from April 1st 1993.* Supplementary General Inspectorate.

Nelson, S. (1997). 'Pastoral Care and Moral Government: Early Nineteenth Century Nursing and Solutions to the Irish Question.' *Journal of Advanced Nursing,* **26,** 6–14.

Nettleton, S. (1995). *The Sociology of Health and Illness.* Cambridge: Polity Press.

Newby, H. (1985). *Green and Pleasant Land? Social Change in Rural England.* London: Hutchinson.

Newman, G. (1939). *The Building of a Nation's Health.* London: Macmillan – now Palgrave Macmillan.

Nightingale, F. (1859). *Notes on Nursing: What It is and What It is Not.* London: Harrison and Sons.

Nightingale, F. (1881). *Trained Nursing for the Sick Poor.* London: Spottiswoode & Co.

North, N. (1997). 'Consumers: Service Users or Citizens?' North and Bradshaw (eds), *Perspectives in Health Care.* Basingstoke: Macmillan – now Palgrave Macmillan.

Oakley, A. (1984). *The Captive Womb: A History of the Medical Care of Pregnant Women.* Oxford: Blackwell.

The Observer (2000). 'Teen Sex Tough Love.' *The Observer,* 27 August, 22.

Oda, D. (1985). 'Community Health Nursing in Innovative School Health Roles and Programmes.' In Archer, S. and Fleshman, R. (eds), *Community Health Nursing,* 3rd edn. Wadsworth, Monterey.

Oppenheim and Harker (1996). *Poverty, the Facts.* London: Child Poverty Action Group.

Orwell, G. (1937). *The Road to Wigan Pier.* London: Gollancz.

Osborn, F. and Whittick, A. (1969). *The New Towns.* London: Leonard Hill.

Osborne, T. (1997). 'Of Health and Statecraft.' In Petersen, A. and Bunton, R. (eds), *Foucault, Health and Medicine.* London: Routledge.

Pahl, R. (1965). *Urbs in Rure.* London: London School of Economics Geographical Papers 2.

Parton, N. (1985). *The Politics of Child Abuse.* Basingstoke: Macmillan – now Palgrave Macmillan.

Pearce, I. and Crocker, L. (1943), reprinted 1985. *The Peckham Experiment: A Study in the Living Structure of Society.* Edinburgh: Scottish Academic Press.

Pearson, G. (1977). *The Deviant Imagination.* London: Macmillan – now Palgrave Macmillan.

Pember Reeves, M. (1913), republished 1979. *Round About a Pound a Week.* London: Virago.

Petchey, R. (1986). 'The Griffiths Reorganisation of the NHS.' *Critical Social Policy,* **17:** 2, 87–101.

Piachaud, D. (1999). 'Progress on Poverty.' *New Economy,* **6:** 3, 154–60.

Policy Studies Institute (1998). *Ethnic Minorities in the Inner City.* York: Joseph Rowntree Foundation Findings 988.

Pollit, C. (1993). *Managerialism and the Public Services,* 2nd edn. Oxford: Basil Blackwell.

Porter, R. (1999). *The Greatest Benefit to Mankind.* London: Fonatana Press.

Porter, S. (1992). 'The Poverty of Professionalisation: A Critical Analysis of Strategies for the Occupational Advancement of Nursing.' *The Journal of Advanced Nursing,* **17,** 720–6.

Potrykus, C. (1989). 'Facing the Challenge of GP Contracts.' *Health Visitor,* **62,** 363–4.

Power, A. (1987). *Property before People: The Management of Twentieth Century Council Housing.* London: Allen and Unwin.

Power, A. (1993). *Hovels to High Rise.* London: Routledge.

Power, C., Manor, O. and Fox, A. (1991). *Health and Class: The Early Years.* London: Chapman Hall.

Price-Waterhouse (1988). *Nurse Retention and Recruitment: A Matter of Priority.* Report on the Factors Affecting the Retention and Recruitment of Nurses Midwives and Health Visitors. Commissioned by the Chairman of Regional Health Authorities in England, Health Boards in Scotland and Health Authorities in Wales, London: Price-Waterhouse.

Price-Waterhouse, Soothill, K., Henry, C. and Kendrick, K. (eds) (1996) *Themes and Perspectives in Nursing.* London: Chapman and Hall.

Radical Statistics Health Group (1991). 'Missing – A Strategy for the Health of the Nation.' *British Medical Journal,* **303**, 299–302.

Radsma, J. (1994). 'Caring and Nursing: A Dilemma.' *Journal of Advanced Nursing,* **20**, 444–9.

Ravetz, A. (1989). 'A View from the Interior.' In Attfield, J. and Kirkham, P. (eds), *A View from the Interior.* London: The Women's Press.

Reverby, S. (1987). 'The Search for the Hospital Yardstick: Nursing and the Rationalisation of Hospital Work.' In Reverby, S. and Rossner, D. (eds), *Health Care in America: Essays in Social History.* Philadelphia: Temple University Press.

Rex, J. and Moore, R. (1967). *Race, Community and Conflict.* London: Oxford University Press for Institute of Race Relations.

Richardson, D. (1993). *Women, Motherhood and Childrearing.* Basingstoke: Macmillan – now Palgrave Macmillan.

Roberts, M. (1991). *Living in a Man Made World.* London: Routledge.

Robinson, J. (1982). *An Evaluation of Health Visiting.* London: Council for the Education and Training of Health Visitors.

Robinson, J. (1992). 'Introduction: Beginning the Study of Nursing Policy.' In Robinson, J., Gray, A. and Elkan, R. (eds), *Policy Issues in Nursing.* Buckingham: Open University Press.

Robinson, J. and Strong, P. M. (1987). *Professional Nursing Advice after Griffiths: An Interim Report.* Coventry: University of Warwick, Nursing Policy Studies Centre.

Roof (1990). Editorial, January–February.

Room, G. (1999). *Social Exclusion, Solidarity and the Challenge of Globalisation.* University of Bath Social Policy Papers 27.

Rose, E., Deakin, N., Abrams, M., Jackson, V., Peston, M., Vanags, A., Cohen, B., Gaiskell, J. and Ward, P. (1969). *Colour and Citizenship.* London: Oxford University Press.

Rowntree Foundation (1995). *Mapping British Society.* Findings Social Research Paper 87. York: Joseph Rowntree Foundation.

Rowntree Foundation (1997). *Changing Mortality Ratios in Local Areas of Britain 1950s–1990s.* Social Policy Research 126. York: Rowntree Foundation.

Rowntree Foundation (1997a). *Private Lives and Public Responses: Lone Parenthood and Future Policy.* Foundations, July. York: Rowntree Foundation.

Sagan, L. (1987). *The Health of Nations.* New York: Basic Books.

Salmon, M., Talashek, M. and Tichy, A. (1988). 'Health for All: A Transnational Model for Nursing.' *International Nursing Review,* **35**: 4, 107–9.

Saraga, E. (1993). 'The Abuse of Children.' In Dallos, R. and McLaughlin, E. (eds), *Social Problems and the Family.* London: Open University Press.

Scottish Executive (1999). *Towards a Healthier Scotland – A White Paper on Health.* Cmnd 4269. Edinburgh: The Stationery Office.

Scottish Office (SO) (1998). *Working Together for a Healthier Scotland.* Edinburgh: Scottish Office.

Scull, A. (1979). *Museums of Madness – The Social Organisation of Insanity in 19th Century England*. London: Allen Lane.

Scull, A. (1993). *The Most Solitary of Afflictions: Madness and Society in Britain 1700–1900*. New Haven, London: Yale University Press.

Scull, A. (1996). 'Asylums, Utopias and Realities.' In Tomlinson, D. and Carrier, J. (eds), *Asylum in the Community*. London: Routledge.

Searl, G. (1971). *The Quest for National Efficiency*. Oxford: Blackwell.

Searle, G. (1976). *Eugenics and Politics in Britain 1900–1914*. London: Leyden Noordholf International.

Shears, M. and Coleman, M. (1999). 'Mental Health Nursing Policy – An Exploratory Qualitative Study of Managers' Opinions.' *Journal of Advanced Nursing*, **29**: 6, 1385–92.

Showalter, E. (1981). 'Florence Nightingale's Feminist Complaint: Women, Religion and Suggestions for Thought.' *Signs*, **6**: 3, 395–412.

Showalter, E. (1989). *The Female Malady: Women, Madness and the English Culture 1830–1980*. London: Virago.

Skellington, R. (1993). 'Homelessness.' In Dallos, R. and Mclaughlin, E. (eds), *Social Problems and the Family*. London: Open University/Sage.

Skidmore, D. (1994). *The Ideology of Community Care*. London: Chapman and Hall.

SMAC and SNMAC (1981). Harding Report.

Smith, D. (1989). ' "Not Getting On, Just Getting By." Changing Prospects in South Birmingham.' In Cooke, P. (ed.), *Localities*. London: Unwin Hyman.

Smith, F. B. (1979). *The People's Health 1830–1910*. London: Croom Helm.

Smith, S. (1989). *The Politics of 'Race' and Residence*. London: Polity Press.

Social Exclusion Unit (1997). *Social Exclusion Unit*. Cabinet Office, London: HMSO.

Social Exclusion Unit (1999). *Truancy and School Exclusion Report*. Cabinet Office, London: HMSO.

Social Exclusion Unit (1999a). *Teenage Pregnancy*. Cabinet Office, London: HMSO.

Social Exclusion Unit (2001). *National Strategy for Neighbourhood Renewal*. London: HMSO.

Social Trends (2000). 30, London: Central Statistical Office.

Spring Rice, M. (1939), reprinted 1981. *Working Class Wives*. London: Virago.

Stacey, M. (1970). *Tradition and Change: A Study of Banbury*. Oxford: Oxford University Press.

Stacey, M. and Davies, C. (1983). *Division of Labour in Child Health Care*. London: ESRC and LSE.

Stedman-Jones, G. (1971). *Out Cast London*. Harmondsworth: Penguin Books.

Stephens, T. (ed.) (1945). *Problem Families: An Experiment in Social Rehabilitation*. Liverpool: Pacifist Service Units.

Stimson, G., Alldritt, L., Dolan, K. and Donaghoe, M. (1989). 'Syringe Exchange Schemes in England and Scotland: Evaluating a New Service for Drug Users.' In Aggleton, P., Hart, G. and Davies, P. (eds), *AIDS, Social Representations, Social Practices*. Lewes: Falmer Press.

Stocks, M. (1960). *A Hundred Years of District Nursing*. London: Allen and Unwin.

Stott, D. (1956). *Unsettled Children and their Families*. London: University of London Press.

Strong, P. and Robinson, J. (1990). *The NHS Under New Management*. Buckingham: Open University Press.

Strong, S. (1996). *Community Care*, **16**: 22, 18–19.

Sutton, F. and Smith, C. (1995). 'Advanced Nursing Practice: New Ideas and New Perspectives.' *Journal of Advanced Nursing*, **21**, 1037–43.

Swenarton, M. (1981). *Homes Fit For Heroes: The Politics and Architecture of Early State Housing in Britain*. London: Heineman.

Symonds, A. (1991). 'Angels and Interfering Busybodies: The Social Construction of Two Occupations'. *Sociology of Health and Illness*, **2**: 3, 249–64.

Symonds, A. (1996). 'Expectant Mothers are Hospital Minded: The Politicisation of Childbirth in Britain in the 1930s.' *Civilisation, Sexuality and Social Life in Historical Context*. Simmelweis University of Medicine, Budapest – Conference papers.

Symonds, A. and Kelly, A. (eds) (1998). *The Social Construction of Community Care*. Basingstoke: Macmillan Press – now Palgrave Macmillan.

Takase, M., Kershaw, E. and Burt, L. (2000). 'Nurse–Environment Misfit and Nursing Practice.' *Journal of Advanced Nursing*, September, 3: 56, 819–26.

Tew, M. (1995). *Safer Childbirth; A Critical History of Maternity Care*. London: Chapman Hall.

Thompson, L. (1988). *An Act of Compromise: An Appraisal of the Effects of the Housing Homeless Persons Act 1977*. London: Shelter.

Timmins, N. (1996). *The Five Giants: A Biography of the Welfare State*. London: Fontana.

Titmus, R. (1979). 'Community Care: Fact or Fiction?' In Titmus, R. (ed.), *Commitment to Welfare*. London: Allen and Unwin.

Townsend, P. (1957). *Family Life of Old People: An Inquiry in East London*. London: Routledge Kegan Paul.

Townsend, P. (1962). *Last Refuge: A Survey of Residential Institutions and Homes for the Aged in England and Wales*. London: Routledge Kegan Paul.

Townsend, P., Davidson, N. and Whitehead, M. (eds) (1988). *The Black Report and the Health Divide*. Harmondsworth: Penguin.

Treasury (2000). *Prudent for a Purpose: Spending Review*. London: HMSO.

Turner, B. (1997). 'From Governmentality to Risk.' In Petersen, A. and Bunton, R. (eds), *Foucault, Health and Medicine*. London: Routledge.

Ungerson, C. (1987). *Policy is Personal: Gender and Informal Care*. London: Routledge Kegan Paul.

United Kingdom Central Council (1986). *Project 2000: A New Preparation for Practice*. London: UKCC.

United Kingdom Central Council (1991). *Report on Proposals for the Future of Community Education and Practice*. London: UKCC.

United Kingdom Central Council (1992). *Code of Professional Conduct for Nurses, Midwives and Health Visitors*, 3rd edn. London: UKCC.

United Kingdom Central Council (1994). *The Future of Professional Practice: The Council's Standards for Specialist Education and Practice Following Registration*. London: UKCC.

United Kingdom Central Council (2001). *Developing Standards and Competencies for Health Visitors*. London: UKCC.

Vaughan, B. (1999). 'Exploring New Roles in Practice.' *Health Service Journal*.

Walby, S. and Greenwell, J. (1994). *Medicine and Nursing: Professions in a Changing Health Service*. London: Sage.

Walkowitz, J. (1982). 'Male Vice and Feminist Virtue: Feminism and the Politics of Prostitution in Nineteenth Century Britain.' *History Workshop*, **13**, 110–29.

Walsh, N. and Gough, P. (1997). *From Profession to Commodity: The Case of Community Nursing*. Unpublished paper.

Waszynski, C. M., Murakami, W. and Lewis, M. (2000). 'Community Care Management. Advanced Practice Nurses as Care Managers.' *Care Management Journal*, Fall, **23**, 148–52.

Warner, M., Longley, M., Gould, E. and Picek, A. (1998). *Healthcare Futures 2010*. Commissioned by the UKCC Education Committee.

Warren, K. S. (1988). 'The Evolution of Selective Primary Health Care.' *Social Science and Medicine*, **26**: 9, 891–8.

Watson, N. (1984). 'Community as a Client.' In Sullivan, J. (ed.), *Directions in Community Health Nursing*. Oxford: Blackwell Scientific.

Webber, I. (1998). 'Professions and School Nursing.' In Symonds, A. and Kelly, A. (eds), *Social Construction of Community Care*. Basingstoke: Macmillan Press – now Palgrave Macmillan.

Webster, C. (1982). 'The Healthy or Hungry Thirties?' *History Workshop*, **13**, 110–29.

Webster, C. (1988). *The Health Services Since the War*. London: HMSO.

Webster, C. (1988). *Problems of Health Care: The NHS before 1957*. London: HMSO.

Webster, C. (1991). *Aneurin Bevan on the National Health Service*. Oxford: Welcome Unit.

Weeks, J. (1981). *Sex, Politics and Society since 1800*. London: Longman.

Weeks, J. (1989). 'AIDS: the Intellectual Agenda.' In Aggleton, P., Hart, G. and Davies, G. (eds), *AIDS Social Representations Social Practices*. Lewes: Falmer Press.

Wellings, K. (1988). 'Perceptions of Risk – Media Treatments of AIDS.' In Aggleton, P. and Homans, H. (eds), *Social Aspects of AIDS*. Lewes: Falmer Press.

Welsh Office (WO) (1997). *Health Gain Targets for Wales*, [DGM97] 50. Welsh Office: Cardiff.

Welsh Office (WO) (1998). *Better Health – Better Wales*. Cardiff: Welsh Office.

Welshman, J. (1996). 'Physical Education and the School Medical Service in England and Wales, 1907–1939.' *Society for the Social History of Medicine*, **9**: 1, 31–45.

White, E. (1993). 'Community Psychiatric Nursing 1980–1990: A Review of Organisation, Education and Practice.' In Booker, C. and White, E. (eds), *Community Psychiatric Nursing: A Research Perspective, vol. 2*. London: Chapman and Hall.

Wilkinson, J. (1998). 'Danger on the Streets: Community Care and Ingratitude.' Symonds, A. and Kelly, A. (eds), *The Social Construction of Community Care*. Basingstoke: Macmillan Press – now Palgrave Macmillan.

Wilkinson, M. (1995). 'Love is not a Marketable Commodity: New Public Management in the British NHS.' *Journal of Advanced Nursing*, **21**, 980–7.

Wilkinson, R. (1996). *Unhealthy Societies*. London: Routledge.

Wilkinson, R. and Davey-Smith, G. (1989). 'Class Mortality Differentials, Income Distribution and Trends in Poverty 1921–1981.' *Journal of Social Policy*, **18**, 307–35.

Williams, C. (1985). 'Population-focused Community Health Nursing and Nursing Administration: A New Synthesis.' In Comi-McCloskey, J. and Kennedy-Grace, H. (eds) *Current Issues in Nursing*, 2nd edn. Boston: Blackwell.

Williams, R. (1975). *The Country and the City*. London: Chatto and Windus.

Williams, R. (1983). *Key Words: Vocabulary of Culture and Society*. London: Fontana.

Wiseman, T. (1989). 'Marginalised Groups and Health Education about HIV and AIDS.' Aggleton, P., Hart, G. and Davies (eds), *AIDS Social Representations Social Practices*. Lewes: Falmer Press.

Wohl, Y. (1983). *Endangered Lives: Public Health in Victorian Britain*. London: Methuen.

Women's Group on Public Welfare (1943). *Our Towns*. Oxford: Oxford University Press.

World Health Organisation (WHO) (1986). *First International Conference on Health Promotion. The Move Towards a New Public Health; Ottawa Charter for Health Promotion*, Ottawa, Nov. 17–21. Ottawa: WHO/Health and Welfare Canada/ Canadian Association for Public Health.

World Health Organisation (WHO) (1986a). *Declaration of Alma Ata. Report of the International Conference on Primary Health Care*. Geneva: WHO/Unicef.

World Health Organisation Europe (WHO) (1984). *Summary Report of the Working Group on Concepts and Principles of Health Promotion*. Copenhagen: WHO Regional Office for Europe.

Youth Justice Board (1999). *Parenting in the Youth Justice Context*.

Zweig, F. (1961). *The Worker in an Affluent Society*. Harmondsworth: Penguin Books.

Index